Cerebral Palsy

Editor

ALOYSIA LEISANNE SCHWABE

PHYSICAL MEDICINE AND REHABILITATION CLINICS OF NORTH AMERICA

www.pmr.theclinics.com

Consulting Editor
SANTOS F. MARTINEZ

February 2020 • Volume 31 • Number 1

ELSEVIER

1600 John F. Kennedy Boulevard • Suite 1800 • Philadelphia, Pennsylvania, 19103-2899

http://www.theclinics.com

PHYSICAL MEDICINE AND REHABILITATION CLINICS OF NORTH AMERICA Volume 31, Number 1
February 2020 ISSN 1047-9651, ISBN 978-0-323-70952-1

Editor: Lauren Boyle
Developmental Editor: Laura Fisher

Reprints. For copies of 100 or more of articles in this publication, please contact the Commercial Reprints Department, Elsevier Inc., 360 Park Avenue South, New York, NY 10010-1710. Tel.: 212-633-3874; Fax: 212-633-3820; E-mail: reprints@elsevier.com.

Physical Medicine and Rehabilitation Clinics of North America (ISSN 1047-9651) is published quarterly by Elsevier Inc., 360 Park Avenue South, New York, NY 10010-1710. Months of issue are February, May, August, and November. Business and Editorial Offices: 1600 John F. Kennedy Blvd., Suite 1800, Philadelphia, PA 19103-2899. Customer Service Office: 3251 Riverport Lane, Maryland Heights, MO 63043. Periodicals postage paid at New York, NY and additional mailing offices. Subscription price per year is $313.00 (US individuals), $633.00 (US institutions), $100.00 (US students), $366.00 (Canadian individuals), $833.00 (Canadian institutions), $100.00 (Canadian students), $429.00 (foreign individuals), $833.00 (foreign institutions), and $210.00 (foreign students). Foreign air speed delivery is included in all *Clinics* subscription prices. All prices are subject to change without notice. **POSTMASTER:** Send address changes to *Physical Medicine and Rehabilitation Clinics of North America*, Customer Service Office: Elsevier Health Sciences Division, Subscription Customer Service, 3251 Riverport Lane, Maryland Heights, MO 63043. **Customer Service: 1-800-654-2452 (US). From outside of the United States, call 314-447-8871. Fax: 314-447-8029. E-mail: JournalsCustomer Service-usa@elsevier.com (for print support); JournalsOnlineSupport-usa@elsevier.com (for online support).**

Physical Medicine and Rehabilitation Clinics of North America is indexed in *Excerpta Medica, MEDLINE/PubMed (Index Medicus), Cinahl,* and *Cumulative Index to Nursing and Allied Health Literature.*

Contributors

CONSULTING EDITOR

SANTOS F. MARTINEZ, MD, MS
Diplomate of the American Academy of Physical Medicine and Rehabilitation, Certificate of Added Qualification Sports Medicine, Assistant Professor, Department of Orthopaedics, Campbell Clinic Orthopaedics, University of Tennessee, Memphis, Tennessee

EDITOR

ALOYSIA LEISANNE SCHWABE, MD
Associate Professor, Departments of Physical Medicine and Rehabilitation and Pediatrics, Baylor College of Medicine, Section Chief/Co-Director of Cerebral Palsy Clinic and Motion Lab, Pediatric Physical Medicine and Rehabilitation, Texas Children's Hospital, Houston, Texas

AUTHORS

ANGELA P. ADDISON, BS
Research Assistant, Department of Neurosurgery, Section of Pediatric Neurosurgery, Baylor College of Medicine, Houston, Texas

AMY F. BAILES, PT, PhD
Division of Occupational Therapy and Physical Therapy, Cincinnati Children's Hospital Medical Center, Cincinnati, Ohio

DOROTHY H. BEAUVAIS, MD
Division of Pediatric Orthopaedic Surgery, Texas Children's Hospital, Assistant Professor of Orthopaedic Surgery, Baylor College of Medicine, Houston, Texas

JOHN BERENS, MD
Assistant Professor, Department of Internal Medicine, Section of Transition Medicine, Baylor College of Medicine, Houston, Texas

DANIEL J. CURRY, MD
Associate Professor, Department of Neurosurgery, Section of Pediatric Neurosurgery, Baylor College of Medicine, Houston, Texas

SALLY A. DiBELLO, MPO, CPO
Assistant Professor of Orthotics and Prosthetics, Baylor College of Medicine School of Health Professions, Prosthetist Orthotist, Hanger Clinic, Houston, Texas

SHANNON M. DiCARLO, MD
Assistant Professor, Division of Neurology and Departmental Neurosciences, Department of Pediatrics, Co-director, Cerebral Palsy Clinic, Baylor College of Medicine, Houston, Texas

ERIC L. DUGAN, PhD
Associate Professor, Department of Orthopedic Surgery, Baylor College of Medicine, Houston, Texas; Texas Children's Hospital, The Woodlands, Texas

ROCHELLE DY, MD
Associate Professor, Physical Medicine and Rehabilitation, Texas Children's Hospital, Houston, Texas

LISA T. EMRICK, MD
Medical Director of Neurogenetics, Assistant Professor, Division of Neurology and Departmental Neurosciences, Department of Pediatrics, Assistant Professor, Department of Human and Molecular Genetics, Baylor College of Medicine, Houston, Texas

DEBORAH GAEBLER-SPIRA, MD
Professor of Pediatrics and Physical Medicine and Rehabilitation, Shirley Ryan Ability Lab, Northwestern University Feinberg School of Medicine, Chicago, Illinois

MARY E. GANNOTTI, PT, PhD
Department of Rehabilitation Sciences, University of Hartford, West Hartford, Connecticut

JOSLYN GOBER, DO
Pediatric Rehabilitation Medicine Fellow, Department of Physical Medicine and Rehabilitation, Baylor College of Medicine, Texas Children's Hospital, Houston, Texas

PAUL H. GROSS
Department of Population Health Sciences, University of Utah, Salt Lake City, Utah

JOHN A. HEYDEMANN, MD
Division of Pediatric Orthopaedic Surgery, Texas Children's Hospital, Assistant Professor of Orthopaedic Surgery, Baylor College of Medicine, Houston, Texas

SUSAN D. HORN, PhD
Adjunct Professor, Health System Innovation and Research Division, Department of Population Health Sciences, University of Utah School of Medicine, Salt Lake City, Utah

EDWARD A. HURVITZ, MD
Department of Physical Medicine and Rehabilitation, Michigan Medicine/University of Michigan, Ann Arbor, Michigan

ANNA O. JESUS, MD
Fellow in Neurodevelopmental and Behavioral Pediatrics, University of Virginia, UVA Neurodevelopmental and Behavioral Pediatrics, Charlottesville, Virginia

MEGAN R. LOMAX, MMS, MPAS, PA-C
Physician Assistant, Orthopedic Surgery, Texas Children's Hospital, Instructor, Orthopedic Surgery, Baylor College of Medicine, Houston, Texas

MAUREEN R. NELSON, MD
Associate Professor, Department of Physical Medicine and Rehabilitation, Baylor College of Medicine, Children's Hospital of San Antonio, San Antonio, Texas

CHRISTIAN NIEDZWECKI, DO
Assistant Professor, H. Ben Taub Department of Physical Medicine and Rehabilitation, Baylor College of Medicine, Texas Children's Hospital, Houston, Texas

CYNTHIA PEACOCK, MD
Associate Professor, Department of Internal Medicine, Section of Transition Medicine, Medical Director of Texas Children's Hospital, Baylor College of Medicine, Transition Medicine Clinic, Houston, Texas

FABIOLA REYES, MD
Pediatric PM&R Fellow, H. Ben Taub Department of Physical Medicine and Rehabilitation, Baylor College of Medicine, Texas Children's Hospital, Houston, Texas

DESIREE ROGE, MD
Associate Professor, Pediatric Rehabilitation Medicine, Seattle Children's Hospital, Department of Physical Medicine and Rehabilitation, University of Washington, Seattle, Washington, USA

KATHERINE M. SCHROEDER, MD
Division of Pediatric Orthopaedic Surgery, Texas Children's Hospital, Assistant Professor of Orthopaedic Surgery, Baylor College of Medicine, Houston, Texas

ALOYSIA LEISANNE SCHWABE, MD
Associate Professor, Departments of Physical Medicine and Rehabilitation and Pediatrics, Baylor College of Medicine, Section Chief/Co-Director of Cerebral Palsy Clinic and Motion Lab, Pediatric Physical Medicine and Rehabilitation, Texas Children's Hospital, Houston, Texas

JEFFREY S. SHILT, MD
Associate Professor, Department of Orthopedic Surgery, Baylor College of Medicine, Houston, Texas; Chief of Community Surgery, Co-Medical Director of Motion Analysis Laboratory, Texas Children's Hospital, The Woodlands, Texas

M. WADE SHRADER, MD
Endowed Chair and Division Chief of Cerebral Palsy, Nemours A.I. duPont Hospital for Children, Wilmington, Delaware

RICHARD D. STEVENSON, MD
Professor of Pediatrics, Head, Division of Neurodevelopmental and Behavioral Pediatrics, University of Virginia School of Medicine, University of Virginia, UVA Neurodevelopmental and Behavioral Pediatrics, Charlottesville, Virginia

SRUTHI P. THOMAS, MD, PhD
Assistant Professor, Departments of Physical Medicine and Rehabilitation and Neurosurgery, Section of Pediatric Neurosurgery, Baylor College of Medicine, Houston, Texas

STEPHANIE TOW, MD
Pediatric Sports Medicine Fellow, Sports Medicine Center, Department of Orthopedics, Children's Mercy Kansas City, Kansas City, Missouri

JILDA N. VARGUS-ADAMS, MD, MSc
Associate Professor, Departments of Pediatrics, and Neurology and Rehabilitation Medicine, University of Cincinnati College of Medicine, Division of Pediatric Rehabilitation Medicine, Cincinnati Children's Hospital Medical Center, Cincinnati, Ohio

CYNTHIA WOZOW, DO
Fellow PGY-5, Department of Physical Medicine and Rehabilitation, Baylor College of Medicine/Texas Children's Hospital, Houston, Texas

ED WRIGHT, MD
Associate Professor of Pediatric Physical Medicine and Rehabilitation, Baylor College of Medicine, Pediatric Physiatrist, Texas Children's Hospital, Houston, Texas

Contents

> Children with cerebral palsy (CP) will be cared for at some point by all pe-
> diatricians and many pediatric subspecialists due to this condition being
> the most common motor disability of childhood. Comprehensive care of
> the child with CP requires individuals with specialized training, and these
> children benefit from an interdisciplinary team approach to care. CP is het-
> erogeneous due to varied causes, which necessitates individualized treat-
> ment plans. The CP specialist must be prepared to support the needs of
> the child with CP holistically and must dialogue regularly with members
> of the team and involve the family in decision-making.

> Cerebral palsy is a clinical diagnosis of a nonprogressive developmental
> disorder of motor impairment. The scope of the diagnosis of cerebral palsy
> has been broadening significantly in recent years to include patients with
> genetic disorders. This article helps clinicians to determine which patients
> would benefit from a thorough genetic/metabolic evaluation and helps to
> delineate an approach for the work-up, with an emphasis on newer tech-
> nologies and the evolving fields of fetal medicine and genetics. It provides
> guidance to providers to assist in clarifying an cause for some patient's
> symptoms.

> Children with cerebral palsy (CP) are at risk of growth and nutrition disor-
> ders. There are numerous challenges to measure and assess growth and
> nutritional status in children with CP. Addressing these challenges is
> imperative, because the consequences of poor growth and malnutrition
> range from decreased bone density, muscle mass, and quality of life to im-
> pacts on intellectual quotient, behavior, attention, social participation,
> healthcare utilization, and health care costs. In addition to discussing ap-
> proaches to assess growth and nutrition, this article examines some of the
> methods of optimizing nutrition and bone health, including when preparing
> for and recovering from surgery.

Scoliosis, hip dysplasia, and other lower extremity deformities are common musculoskeletal pathology found in patients with cerebral palsy. Imaging studies allow for an improved identification of patients with these issues, help to understand the pathology, and aid in planning treatment strategies. Most of these deformities are visualized using plain radiographic techniques. Occasionally, as in the case of preoperative planning, advanced imaging, such as computerized topography and MRI, can be used for additional information. This article provides insight into the various imaging techniques for these musculoskeletal issues and aids in better care for patients with cerebral palsy.

Identifying the subtypes of hypertonia is becoming increasingly important. Treatment strategies, including tone-modulating surgical interventions, medication type and dosing, and chemodenervation, may differ depending on the type of hypertonia present. It is important to delineate how hypertonia interferes with function and quality of life so that the appropriate intervention can be selected at the right time. Outcomes of treatment depend heavily on clear communication of goals. Botulinum toxin should not be used in isolation but as an adjunct to rehabilitation modalities.

▶ Video content accompanies this article at http://www.pmr.theclinics. com.

Maintenance of upright posture and gait mobility is frequently a goal in supporting children with cerebral palsy (CP). Ankle-foot orthoses (AFOs) can play an important role in normalizing gait function in this population. Properly designed orthotic interventions consider common ankle and foot deformities, range-of-motion limitations, and natural history of CP. Successful AFO prescription often requires interaction with complementary interventions such as physical therapy, spasticity management, and/or orthopedic management. Recognizing the impact of plantar flexion contractures and the effects of footwear on AFO alignment is key to effective orthotic management of gait dysfunction in children with CP.

This article overviews the surgical options for hypertonia management in cerebral palsy, both spasticity and dystonia. We review the history and use of intrathecal baclofen. We contrast its use with the indications for selective dorsal rhizotomy and review how it is the optimal technique to lower tone in the ambulatory spastic diplegic patient with cerebral palsy. This article reviews the advent of deep brain stimulation, with an emphasis on selection criteria and expected outcomes in this population. The article reviews the principles and use of selective peripheral neurotomy as it is applied to focal spasticity not requiring systemic tone reduction.

Gait abnormalities in cerebral palsy are complex and difficult to accurately characterize. Clinical gait analysis shows the prerequisite components of a clinical test to aid in the treatment planning for patients with cerebral palsy. Clinical gait analysis can be used to distinguish between different levels of impairment, can be used to monitor progress and outcomes, and is beginning to show promise for prediction of postsurgical outcomes. Clinical gait analysis can also provide important and relevant information for treatment planning, enhance the likelihood of positive outcomes, and reduce the number of negative outcomes.

Smaller, smarter, more portable rehabilitation technology has the potential to improve the ability of individuals with cerebral palsy to perform activities and increase participation. Robotics and virtual reality may improve movement by maximizing exercise dose, providing feedback, and motivating users. Augmentative and alternative communication technology is facilitating communication. Robots can help with self-care and provide encouragement and instruction in rehabilitation programs. Mobile applications can provide education and resources. Conducting high-quality research to validate technological advances in our field has been a major focus of researchers and advocacy groups.

Care and research in childhood cerebral palsy (CP) continue to evolve. As our understanding of CP grows more nuanced, so grows our need to describe function, activities, challenges, adaptations of children with CP. In CP, robust means of measuring outcomes are vital to understanding utility of treatments. Research must accurately measure meaningful constructs of children with CP as a reliable ruler to establish if interventions produce useful effects. This article addresses the challenges of outcome measurement in CP, current status of outcome measurement in CP, and issues of understanding change in childhood CP.

 Video content accompanies this article at http://www.pmr.theclinics.com.

Adaptive sports and recreation have an important role in the lifestyle of individuals with cerebral palsy (CP). This article discusses the history of adaptive sports and the benefits of adaptive sports and recreation. Barriers and medical challenges are also thoroughly discussed, including common musculoskeletal issues, methods to prevent musculoskeletal injury, pain, fatigue, maximal exertion, and other medical comorbidities and illness. The role of health care providers such as physiatrists is emphasized to provide support to individuals with CP who either are interested in starting exercise or a sport or are already an athlete.

John Berens, Cynthia Wozow, and Cynthia Peacock

The transition from pediatric-based to adult-based health care is often difficult, especially for individuals with chronic illness or developmental disabilities, such as cerebral palsy. This article describes the current state of health care transition, focusing on some of the elements that contribute to the complexity of this challenging life period, including: changes to health care insurance, medicolegal considerations and options for supported decision making, discussions about vocations and related barriers and resources, and important psychosocial issues faced by many patients with cerebral palsy. Evidence-based processes and practices are described that can help facilitate health care transition planning and improve outcomes.

Megan R. Lomax and M. Wade Shrader

Orthopedic conditions are common in adults with cerebral palsy (CP). Although CP is argued to be a nonprogressive condition of the brain, the musculoskeletal components tend to worsen and deteriorate over time leading to chronic pain, function limitation, and a decline in mobility. Orthopedic care of adults with CP has not been well documented in the literature. This article describes the common orthopedic conditions in adults with CP and discusses who should perform orthopedic surgery on adults.

Edward A. Hurvitz, Paul H. Gross, Mary E. Gannotti, Amy F. Bailes, and Susan D. Horn

Registries are a powerful tool for clinical research. Clinical registries for cerebral palsy can aid in comparative effectiveness research, especially using the practice-based evidence model. The Cerebral Palsy Research Network (CPRN) was initiated in 2014 as a patient-centered, multidisciplinary registry. The leadership group initiated a 4-stage participatory action research process: listen, reflect, plan/analyze, and take action. CPRN also joined with CP NOW, an advocacy group, to create a research agenda for cerebral palsy. With more than 20 centers and growing, CPRN hopes to generate evidence for developing best practices and measure their implementation and impact for individuals with cerebral palsy throughout North America.

PHYSICAL MEDICINE AND REHABILITATION CLINICS OF NORTH AMERICA

SERIES OF RELATED INTEREST

Orthopedic Clinics
Clinics In Sports Medicine

VISIT THE CLINICS ONLINE!
Access your subscription at:
www.theclinics.com

Foreword

A Challenge for All

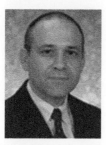

Santos F. Martinez, MD, MS
Consulting Editor

There are many facets to consider for the clinician treating cerebral palsy. These range from preventive efforts and identification of risk factors for prospective mothers to early intervention by the rehabilitation team to address strategies for delayed developmental milestones. There are a number of additional congenital and/or acquired conditions, which include not only neurodevelopmental challenges but also less obvious comorbidities, which may be multiorgan in nature. Vigilance and thoroughness to provide basic nutritional support, multispecialty assessments, and a cohesive plan with family input are paramount.

Although there is a tendency for some to consider cerebral palsy a static condition with well-defined pathology, each patient is different, and there are many phases that the patient, family, and clinician must adapt to with ever-evolving strategies through time to optimize their function and integration into society.

Santos F. Martinez, MD, MS
American Academy of Physical
Medicine and Rehabilitation
Campbell Clinic Orthopaedics
Department of Orthopaedics
University of Tennessee
Memphis, TN 38104, USA

E-mail address:
smartinez@campbellclinic.com

Preface

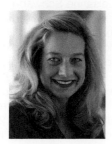

Aloysia Leisanne Schwabe, MD
Editor

This issue of *Physical Medicine and Rehabilitation Clinics of North America* on cerebral palsy incorporates what for many of us is an example of what medicine at its finest can do in making a difference for a child with a lifelong condition. Individuals with different backgrounds and expertise work together to advance a child and their family along a continuum that includes anticipatory guidance, partnering to identify goals, and support to the patient and family through the ups and downs of diagnosis, treatment, and aging. I have been privileged to have a family member myself with cerebral palsy, who will benefit immensely from the expertise available today as a result of the efforts of all of the different disciplines that contribute to care of these individuals.

The contributors to this issue of *Physical Medicine and Rehabilitation Clinics of North America* share in common a passion for caring for children with cerebral palsy. The work is interdisciplinary, and we seek out collaboration and support in pursuing excellence in advancing their care forward. This issue touches on current and new management philosophies, but what is so exciting about this population is that novel treatment concepts and ways of measuring impact on function and quality of life are being investigated constantly. Advocacy efforts continue to draw attention to this patient group, and we celebrate the lives of our patients touched by health care providers, community support organizations, and researchers. Having a lifelong condition creates strong bonds between parents and their supporters. Due to the prevalence of cerebral palsy, it is inevitable that a physician or therapist has not personally been touched by the courageous determination demonstrated by a patient and their family members.

I have had the privilege of working alongside excellent clinicians but also friends in striving to make a difference in the lives of the children we treat. I am incredibly

Phys Med Rehabil Clin N Am 31 (2020) xv–xvi
https://doi.org/10.1016/j.pmr.2019.11.001
1047-9651/20/© 2019 Published by Elsevier Inc.

pmr.theclinics.com

grateful to my patients, who have taught me many lessons over the years and who continue to amaze me.

Aloysia Leisanne Schwabe, MD
Departments of Physical Medicine
and Rehabilitation and Pediatrics
Baylor College of Medicine
Pediatric Physical Medicine
and Rehabilitation
Texas Children's Hospital
6701 Fannin Street
Mark Wallace Tower, Suite 1280
Houston, TX 77030, USA

E-mail address:
aschwabe@bcm.edu

Comprehensive Care in Cerebral Palsy

Aloysia Leisanne Schwabe, MD[a,b,c,*]

KEYWORDS

- Cerebral • palsy • Comprehensive care • Care coordination • Family centered care

KEY POINTS

- Cerebral palsy (CP) management requires knowledgeable specialists and interdisciplinary teams.
- CP is a heterogeneous condition due to varied causes, neuroanatomical correlates, and degrees of severity, which necessitates individualized treatment plans.
- A family centered approach with care coordination decreases parental or caregiver burden.
- There is a greater emphasis today on recommending medical and surgical treatments in CP that are evidence based.
- The CP specialist must be prepared to support the needs of the child with CP holistically and must dialogue regularly with members of the team and involve the family in decision-making.

Cerebral palsy (CP) is the most common motor disability of childhood, and despite technological advancements in medicine, the prevalence of CP has not decreased in developing countries in part due to life-preserving measures now available for the largest subset of children with CP, those who are born prematurely.[1] CP is defined as "a group of permanent disorders of the development of movement and posture, causing activity limitation, that are attributed to non-progressive disturbances that occurred in the developing fetal or infant brain. The motor disorders of CP are often accompanied by disturbances of sensation, perception, cognition, communication, and behavior, by epilepsy; and by secondary musculoskeletal problems.[2]" This expanded definition published in 2006 followed an international workshop where discussion took place about including common impairments and comorbidities observed in CP in the definition as well as its resultant impact on function. Following are the most important criteria to be met when making this clinical diagnosis: (1) motor involvement

[a] Department of Physical Medicine and Rehabilitation, Baylor College of Medicine, Houston, TX, USA; [b] Department of Pediatrics, Baylor College of Medicine, Houston, TX, USA; [c] Pediatric Physical Medicine and Rehabilitation, Texas Children's Hospital, 6701 Fannin Street, Suite 1280, Houston, TX 77030, USA
* 6701 Fannin Street, Suite 1280, Houston, TX 77030.
E-mail address: aschwabe@bcm.edu

Phys Med Rehabil Clin N Am 31 (2020) 1–13
https://doi.org/10.1016/j.pmr.2019.09.012
1047-9651/20/© 2019 Published by Elsevier Inc.
pmr.theclinics.com

must always present, (2) the timing of the insult is early in brain development in the perinatal/infant period, and (3) the course is nonprogressive from a neurologic standpoint. The cause of CP is very diverse, the neuroanatomical findings on imaging also correlating with the clinical phenotype are also varied, and degrees of involvement range from mild to severe, all resulting in different clinical presentations. All of these factors contribute to children having different functional levels. Two children with similar CP phenotypes due to similar causes may then ultimately have different courses due to the additional role of personal and environmental factors and the interplay of other existing medical comorbidities.

When discussing children with CP among care providers, it is desirable to use a common language that immediately conveys the motor abilities of the child from a functional standpoint. The Gross Motor Functional Classification System (GMFCS) was designed to better describe CP involvement and functional mobility taking into consideration the child's age. It effectively communicates both in writing and with visual depictions how independent a child is for mobility and their various needs for physical aids and supports. Over time the GMFCS has been shown to be valid, and assessments of its use with clinicians and parents show good interobserver reliability.[3] The expanded and revised version of the GMFCS now includes adolescents with CP up to age of 18 years and is designed to incorporate the concepts of participation outlined by the International Classification of Functioning, Disability, and Health (ICF). It has been translated into many different languages and is available to download at no cost from the CanChild Website.[4] Children with CP with GMFCS I and II status who are the least involved can ambulate independently, and often a child with GMFCS I status may not be readily observed to have CP when interacting with his or her peers. Children in categories III to IV progressively require more assistance although a child in the GMFCS IV category may be able to drive a power mobility device on their own. GMFCS V children are considered dependent on others or customized equipment for their mobility and need postural supports. As GMFCS level increases, so does the number of comorbidities that are present. There are many other classification systems and functional scales that describe the child with CP. Because all children with CP have some degree of motor disability, the GMFCS is referenced most commonly in literature across various subspecialties.

Because CP is heterogeneous, children with this condition deserve individualized yet comprehensive care, for example, the child with mild diparetic CP who has motor delays with an abnormal gait, spasticity, and impaired balance, but who is independent for mobility and activities of daily living with normal communication skills and cognition without any significant medical comorbidities. This child's care over the years may require more input from specialists who are experts in spasticity management/functional anatomy or the musculoskeletal consequences of CP such as physical therapists, physiatrists, neurosurgeons, and orthopedic surgeons. The child likely will be considered overall healthy and probably will only have hospitalizations related to elective procedures. This is in contrast to the medically complex child with quadriparetic CP with epilepsy, prominent dyskinesias, dysarthria, dysphagia and dysmotility with a gastrostomy tube, recurrent respiratory illnesses, pain from a subluxed hip, and dependence on others for assistance with activities of daily living (ADLs) and mobility due to severe hypertonicity and global weakness. This child will have many more specialists and communication will be ever more challenging in order to facilitate decision-making and to prioritize care with the family's ongoing input. Although both of these children are different, they are best served in programs that emphasize comprehensive care tailored to the individual needs of the child and with CP specialists who have a holistic approach to care, are knowledgeable about CP-associated conditions and scientifically sound available treatment options, and who are part of an interdisciplinary team dedicated to optimizing health and quality of life for those who have this condition. The team members observing these two different children may overlap somewhat, but a CP specialist should follow-up both children closely and help to direct their care. CP specialists should also be immersed in educational activities that allow them to provide comprehensive care in areas that complement their primary specialty in order to participate in anticipatory guidance and to help the family weigh their options especially when considering surgeries.

CP care requires a proactive approach looking for issues these children may experience and being able to recognize when a child is not reaching his/her potential in terms of health and function. Often times CP clinics are found in pediatric teaching hospitals affiliated with an academic institution where clinics are designed to meet the needs of all patients with CP, but especially the very involved child. Community pediatricians now have more resources today in managing children with CP, and there is no excuse for a general provider to counsel a family that the child's situation is unfortunate but without offering care recommendations to promote optimal health and to prevent further disability. Watching and waiting years before referring the child for evaluation to a specialist can be detrimental, as early therapeutic interventions can harness opportunities for progress related to neuroplasticity.[5] Still today children occasionally present for evaluation in our CP clinics who have had no interventions for their hypertonia, who are malnourished, and have already developed severe contractures and deformities, which supports the premise that not all caregivers especially in the community are trained to support these children and that ongoing education is needed. In addition to providing holistic medical care, CP clinics provide education on updated practice guidelines and have local and national resources available for families for supports in the home, school, and community (See the Appendix). Social workers, nutritionists, and therapists are frequently embedded in these specialty clinics as well. Nowadays, most pediatricians readily refer to specialty programs whether this is under the direction of specialists such as physiatrists or developmental pediatricians where they know the child will be cared for comprehensively and all aspects of their health will be optimized.

An additional resource available to the most involved subset of the CP population now are complex care pediatricians who are based in clinics that focus on caring for children with chronic illnesses and conditions that place them at risk for medical deterioration or complications. These children are frequently described as fragile and have dependence on technology. The term "children with medical complexity" (CMC) refers to any child who has

1. Intensive hospital- and/or community-based service need,
2. Reliance on technology, polypharmacy, and/or home care or congregate care to maintain a basic quality of life,
3. Risk of frequent and prolonged hospitalizations, which leads to high health resource utilization, and
4. An elevated need for care coordination.[6]

At the authors' institution, they have a strong, collaborative relationship with the complex care clinic and now have a physiatrist within the clinic to aid in seeing children who use this clinic as a medical home and who are trach/ventilatory dependent to minimize visits that often require ambulance transportation. Complex care pediatricians also participate in providing hospitalist services for these same children when they are admitted and facilitate the transition back to home. A medical home with complex care pediatricians is an excellent option for families where their child's condition warrants lengthier visits with a pediatrician trained to provide care to the disabled child who has numerous medical problems and care-giving issues to be addressed at each visit. Ideally this primary care model would extend into the community, but balancing supply and demand of complex care pediatricians means many remain located at a centrally based tertiary children's hospital. Initiatives are in place for pediatric and adult primary care providers of complex patients to host interested community providers and to use telemedicine to add support and training so that the community providers are comfortable providing this type of care and the family can have access to a primary care provider closer to their home. Most complex care clinics have entrance criteria, which sometimes require a patient to have 3 or more chronic conditions and a minimum number of subspecialists involved in the care of the child as well as technology dependence. Therefore, children with CP who are more mobile in the GMFCS categories of I to III with fewer comorbidities will often be followed by a community pediatrician and rely on a specialty CP clinic/program for their CP specific care. Medically complex patients who live far away and out of necessity prefer a pediatrician close to home for acute issues also are followed-up in the authors' specialty CP clinic where care coordination is supported. The common thread where children are followed regularly by a CP specialist is very important, as preventative measures, treatments, and condition-specific counseling are necessary to manage issues that may affect school performance, independence with mobility and ADLs, and participation in day-to-day activities outside of the home and school. With guidance from the CP clinic team, a plan can be put in place to promote healthy habits, manage hypertonia, and to avoid or limit the musculoskeletal complications that naturally occur related to growth such as contracture formation and musculoskeletal deformity that can result in pain, decreased activity, and additional loss of function and disability. Care coordination is critically important in both settings, the CP clinic and complex care clinic, in order for the child to receive comprehensive care, and often times this is supported by care coordinators and social workers. Even when these disciplines work with the family directly, frontline providers including physicians and advanced practice providers still spend considerable time coordinating care for these children that is nonreimburseable.[7] This may include dialogue with other providers, the patient's therapists and school, and writing letters or completing applications on that patient's behalf. A navigator is also tremendously helpful to assist families through a complicated system where services are spread across a large geographic area and not always consolidated at one location.

Children who are establishing care in a CP clinic should have a comprehensive evaluation including birth and family history or pertinent history that contributes to causality when possible, examination, and diagnostic workup including neuroimaging in the form of MRI. Imaging can support acquired insults as seen in prematurity, hypoxic-ischemic encephalopathy, and stroke but also can reveal migrational defects and malformations. Septo-optic dysplasia is an example of a brain malformation resulting in CP but with common comorbidities of visual disturbances and endocrine abnormalities warranting evaluations with ophthalmology and endocrinology, respectively, knowing the associated comorbidities expected based on imaging help to guide additional evaluations that may affect treatment. Similarly, specifying with greater accuracy the predominant movement abnormality present in the child with CP and confirming a neuroanatomic correlate improves confidence in that patient's responsiveness to treatments aimed at a particular form of hypertonia such as spasticity versus dystonia.[8] To help improve the consistency in using terminology describing various forms of hypertonia, a taskforce was also formed with representation from varied specialties to better define spasticity, dystonia, and other forms of dyskinesias.[9]

The Hypertonia Assessment Tool is also helpful for differentiating between spasticity and dystonia and can be performed quickly in an office setting.[10] If clinicians and researchers alike can use a common set of definitions for describing with better accuracy the types of hypertonia they are observing and feeling on physical examination, then the collective outcomes after a specific intervention tailored to that patient subgroup based on the movement or hypertonia type has greater meaning.

It is important to recognize that some children initially diagnosed as having CP without a clear explanation by history and supporting imaging will eventually be determined to have other conditions that may be inherited. With any neurologic regression or worsening of tone without a clear explanation, repeat imaging and additional studies are warranted, as other conditions that may present at an early age appearing static may turn out to be progressive. This is most commonly accomplished through a neurologist or geneticist (or a "neurogeneticist"). If the child has a progressive course with neurologic deterioration or a genetic syndrome known to have stepwise decline over time is discovered, then the cerebral diagnosis is no longer appropriate. Mimics of CP include spinal dysraphism/occult spinal cord injuries, dopa-responsive dystonia, hereditary spastic paraparesis, and glutaric aciduria to name a few.[11] The role of genetics in CP is increasing and is covered more in depth in a subsequent chapter in this issue. Of note, with a greater emphasis on obtaining genetic testing when there is not a clear causal relationship established to explain a static CP phenotype, there is a growing number of CP cases now with identified genetic mutations. Because genetic testing is more commonplace in the investigation of children presenting with CP, there has been debate over whether these cases should be reclassified once a genetic abnormality is confirmed. The present line of thinking from most clinicians and researchers is that a child with a genetic abnormality but static course that meets the definition for CP should remain included in the CP cohort in order to preserve their access to services and specialized care and programs. In addition, removing these cases could have negative implications from an epidemiologic standpoint.[12]

There are many different medical comorbidities experienced by children with CP. Some are frequently recognized/investigated and then treated, whereas others are not considered due to the lack of obvious physical symptoms and signs or in some cases due to the provider's lack familiarity with this patient population or time limitations in a busy practice to address issues not raised as areas of concern by the parent. Common comorbidities include epilepsy, intellectual disability, failure to thrive, and spasticity/hypertonia and the more severe end of the spectrum of hip and spine deformities being hip dislocation and scoliosis. Some medical issues will be identified during routine pediatric screening administered to all children, such as identifying hearing deficits, but still these are occasionally missed. Conditions that are less frequently recognized and warrant attention and treatment are shown in **Box 1**.

Some basic caveats of CP care should also be noted:

- Pain in CP is frequently present and not recognized. Children with CP often times cannot communicate effectively and pain can present in other ways such as irritability and changes in eating and sleep patterns. Tools for assessing pain in the child with more involved CP who is nonverbal are less than ideal. In many instances, systematically inquiring about these changes in daily routine and asking probing questions about pain is necessary in addition to a thorough examination. There is some evidence to support the use of intrathecal baclofen for relief of pain related to hypertonia.[13]

Box 1
Frequently underdiagnosed or unrecognized medical comorbidities in cerebral palsy

Growth Disturbances	Visual Disturbances without Obvious Strabismus
Premature or delayed puberty	Dysphagia with silent aspiration
Dysmenorrhea	Dysmotility
Obstructive/central apnea	Gastroesophageal reflux disease (GERD)
Impaired cough	Osteopenia/vitamin D deficiency
Urinary retention/dyssynergia	Pain
Autonomic nervous system instability	Depression/anxiety
Myelopathy	Spondylolisthesis
Skin breakdown/decubiti	Nonaccidental trauma

- When reports of spasticity worsening are relayed by caregivers, sources of noxious stimuli that could be responsible for the change in tone should be investigated such as GERD, hip subluxation, skin injury/decubiti, and constipation. Children with CP do not rapidly worsen to a "new baseline." If a child with CP has more than a relatively short period of time, a significant decline in function, worsening of tone, or cognitive status change, then this warrants investigation of underlying causes or consideration of alternative diagnoses.
- Children with CP can develop uncommon medical conditions despite having CP. Signs and symptoms of rarer conditions should not always be attributed to the more common explanation readily available because it occurs in CP. An example would be a child with CP who develops inflammatory bowel disease in the setting of slow transit constipation.

For a comprehensive review of medical comorbidities in CP, the reader is also directed to a dedicated chapter on this topic in a prior issue of Clinics of North America focused on CP.[14]

Fortunately, the optimization of health of children with CP is now receiving greater attention, as more and more surgical programs are putting into place indications, conferences, and preoperative clearance assessments with nutritionists, pulmonary specialists, and anesthesiologists to ensure that the child is optimally ready for elective surgery from a health perspective. Additional evaluations by cardiologists and hematologists may be needed when the child also has a history of a congenital heart disease and/or arrhythmia or bleeding disorder, respectively. These additional steps are resulting in improved patient selection and outcomes.

Not all children with CP have access to the same resources. Initially, where the child is hospitalized in the perinatal period or seen for medical appointments may determine what resources the family is given. Not all children at risk for CP are seen in a neonatal developmental follow-up clinic or by specialists performing a detailed neuromusculoskeletal examination. Before discharge from a neonatal intensive care unit, children will be referred frequently to Early Childhood Intervention (ECI), but access to services through this federal program may be limited depending on where the child lives and how many other children are being served by that program in the area of coverage. If the ECI program is not able to staff a referral at all for a particular discipline of therapy or at the desired frequency, private therapies in a home health- or clinic-based setting can be established. The complexities of coverage for therapies in different settings is beyond the scope of this article, but home health therapy is usually reserved for children who are too medically fragile to transport out of the home (some potential negative impact on health could occur—ie, excessive fatigue, risk for infectious or respiratory complications). At age 3 years, the child can be evaluated for enrollment in a public preschool for children with disabilities program or similar named entity. As expected, some of the programs are more robust than others; parents may elect to wait until the child is older to enroll in public school based on program components including class demographics (whether their child is similar to peers), staff to student ratios, and available adaptive equipment. Ideally, public school are mandated by law to provide education in the least restrictive environment, but often times children are not placed in appropriate classroom settings with proper supports. Some school districts also do not have the ability to diversify a curriculum for a child who is relatively cognitively spared but nonverbal, either by choice or unfortunately due to a lack of recognition of that child's abilities. CP specialists in this case can advocate for the child to have an assistive technology evaluation. Also there is a common misperception among parents and some providers that school systems in the United States must provide regular therapy services. They are in fact required to provide therapy services that are educationally relevant, but this statement has wide room for interpretation. Some public school systems provide excellent academic supports, provide therapy services on a regular basis with a focus on functional goals, and provide equipment specific to that child's needs and train staff appropriately; however, others sometimes fail to provide basic access for children with disabilities and do not make their education a priority. It is therefore important to ascertain what the child's classroom environment is like, what attention and level of instruction that child is receiving, what is being addressed at school by different therapy disciplines, and the frequency of treatments occurring. Parents should be educated on their rights when working with public school systems and in some cases they will need extra help in the form of advocacy. Having the parent sign a consent in order to obtain a copy of an Individualized Education Plan and Admission, Review, and Dismissal meeting documents can be very helpful when there seems to be a discrepancy in what the child is capable of doing academically and what is being provided in terms of instruction. These will also describe frequency of therapy services and accommodations in place. Involving a developmental pediatrician and/or neuropsychologist to evaluate the child is also advisable to aid in formally testing a child with CP who appears to be in a curriculum that is either too rigorous or that is not challenging enough. These specialists also are able to diagnose attention-related disorders and learning disabilities that may require a different instructional approach in order for the child with CP to be successful in reaching their academic potential.

Therapy services are a mainstay of CP treatment. Some children receive all of their therapy services through the school system especially in the case of limited access to clinic-based services or home health services due to transportation, distance, or a caregiver being a single parent with limited options for scheduling. A therapist's knowledge about CP treatments may be robust especially if they participate in CP-specific organizations such as the American Academy of Cerebral Palsy and Developmental Medicine (AACPDM) or limited depending on training and experience. The CP specialist often has therapists on site during clinic visits or available to meet with the patient and family that day that can help fill in gaps where education is needed. Therapy is important for focusing on areas for improvement and aiding the family with setting realistic and appropriate goals. Communication between the treating therapist and the prescribing physician is of upmost importance so that the family is confident that treatments and plans incorporating therapy are jointly recommended and there is collaboration when barriers to progress are reached. Even children who function more independently can benefit from episodic therapy updates to focus on age-appropriate, specific goals and optimizing function so that participation can increase.

These same higher-functioning children may end up with musculoskeletal deformities during periods of rapid growth if anticipatory guidance is not presented and reinforced. A shift in how therapy is delivered is now occurring, which places greater importance on the child's functioning and participation with less of a focus on specific impairments again in alignment with the ICF model.

More involved children with CP with multiple comorbidities are clearly at higher risk for medical complications such as aspiration or community-acquired pneumonia, fragility fractures, decubiti, and severe musculoskeletal deformities. There are routine health maintenance and preventative care pediatric guidelines published tailored to the age of the child. With CP, these same guidelines apply but the developmental stage of the child may lag behind, so counseling regarding expectations of behavior or independence with ADLs or mobility for a particular age group may not be applicable. Some parents benefit from visual diagrams in developmental tools outlining where the child with CP is in different spheres and how they are changing over time to illustrate that "catching up" in all areas may not be possible. Although some children do change GMFCS levels over time, many do not. Discussions should also take place regarding the cognitive abilities of the child over repeated visits so that parents are not surprised to learn that their child has deficits in certain areas especially when this could lead to frustrations and challenges in the academic setting. Cognitive limitations and impaired executive functioning may also affect the ability of the teen to make independent decisions and to direct their care, which may be a difficult subject to broach, but this is a very necessary conversation to have. A very nice compilation of routine pediatric care at age intervals combined with CP-specific guidelines is available from Seattle Children's hospital.[15] It also was developed with input from families and specifically references family involvement in decision making. Ultimately the goal is that children with CP are receiving thorough and evidence-based care tailored to their particular situation and in the context of that family's preferences and values. International organizations such as AACPDM have also worked on publishing care pathways to help make recommendations with expert input and based on available research. There are four existing pathways at the time of this publication, including hip surveillance, dystonia, sialorrhea, and osteoporosis.[16] Awareness, for example, of the need for CP hip screening has increased tremendously due to ongoing discussions and instructional courses at national meetings on this topic, publications about the effectiveness or lack of effectiveness of various interventions, and publications of guidelines. Families can learn about these initiatives also through parent forums, Websites with educational materials/factsheets, and via health care providers who maintain a current knowledge of the latest treatment recommendations and supporting evidence for these interventions. Lists of available Website resources are included in the Appendix.

Although some guidelines and treatments are very easy to embrace by most providers who care for children with CP, there will continue to be differences in opinion on the efficacy, the relative benefit/risk profile, and the timing of certain interventions. This applies to therapy programs, medical management and surgeries and complementary medicine. The CP specialist needs to partner with family members as they explore options for treatment and to actively listen to the older child's desires and concerns when considering interventions that may be very time consuming or involve significant risk such as surgery. Today, more than ever, parents are receiving information from numerous directions, and it may be difficult for them to sort out facts from fiction especially when they are hopeful for a treatment that will make dramatic differences in their child's function. All too often, the promise of rapid improvement or dramatic restoration of damaged neural circuitry combined with anecdotal accounts of benefit lures families into considering treatments and procedures that lack supportive evidence and long-term follow-up. A popular intervention today in lieu of muscle lengthenings where the surgeon can visualize what is being cut is percutaneous lengthenings that are irreversible and typically not combined with osteotomies and foot reconstructions that are necessary to address lever arm dysfunction. There has been a shift in practice to evaluating children for single-event multilevel surgery to address numerous contributing impairments all at once surgically and consolidating a rehabilitation course often preceded by 3-dimensional motion analysis. The concern with "percs" is that there is little data available to support the procedure's efficacy long term.[17] Ultimately many of these children still require multilevel surgery to address their rotational problems, stiff knee gait, and foot deformities down the road. Selective dorsal rhizotomy (SDR) is also performed with different surgical approaches anatomically, and different degrees of percentages of nerve root sectioning are performed. Parents, although, may not appreciate the nuances of how one orthopedic or neurosurgical procedure may vary in technique despite having the same general terminology used to name the operation with greater weight placed on peer recommendation. This phenomenon of social media playing a larger role in the dissemination of anecdotal accounts of benefit and its role in social support and networking when deciding on treatments for children with CP is uptrending with SDR being an example.[18] CP remains a very heterogeneous condition, and some children will show resilience and change for the better in some gait parameters with varied surgical techniques because their underlying strength and selective motor control are better than others. This is in contrast to children with unrecognized weakness, patterned responses, and dyskinesias who may do poorly from a gait perspective after popularized treatments such as "percs" and selective dorsal rhizotomy. There are concerns also that "percs" may result in ultimately accelerating worsening of anterior pelvic tilt when hamstrings are overlengthened and the development of crouch that in the short term may not be appreciated by the family and treating therapists. A CP practitioner must be able to speak to the potential benefits and risks of various medical and surgical treatments for the CP population in general but also point out considerations that are specific to each individual child. Of course the mantra that should be clearly communicated is do no harm, and if a potential treatment could be detrimental to the child's functioning either due to the treatment itself or the child's or family's inability to comply with postoperative recommendations then this should be discussed thoroughly. There are practical considerations to discuss with parents when pursuing any surgical treatments that can include costs due to travel-related expenses and time away from work; time requirements especially if a postoperative rehabilitation stay is advised; and a need to plan for postoperative restrictions, greater difficulty mobilizing the patient, and pain management.

CP research continues to mature, and comparative effectiveness trials are also necessary. The work of individuals such as Iona Novak, OT, for example has also focused on critically appraising CP treatments to ascertain if certain treatments are well supported scientifically.[19] Additional research endeavors must continue focusing on identifying which patient characteristics make an individual more responsive to a particular treatment than others. Personalized or precision medicine is designed to match the most effective treatments to those patients who are "profiled" to benefit most.

CP care inevitably will include fielding questions about popular therapy interventions, procedures that promise rapid improvements in function and minimal risk and recovery time, and specifically stem cell therapies, as it is expected that parents hope that one day there will be readily available "restorative" or curative treatments.

The challenge with many therapy programs advertising superior results with either a proprietary approach or use of specialized equipment is that the data to support better outcomes are lacking. Surgeries have also become popularized, which are performed in high volumes with known detrimental outcomes and no long-term published data to support the specific techniques used. These are both examples where the catch-phrase "quantity does not equal quality" applies in hopes that continued dissemination of information through a scientific approach will encourage cautious optimism but with greater scrutiny on the consumer's part when choosing a particular path to follow. Lastly, although there are exciting advances in the arena of stem cell research, there is still much work to be done before stem cell therapy for CP is considered efficacious and safe. It is concerning that growth of stem cell treatment centers has exponentially occurred and stem cell "tourism" continues to prey on the hopes and dreams of individuals with loved ones who have a variety of neurologic disorders who are willing to sacrifice time and money when they are sometimes only delivered dramatic promises and assured that there is little to no risk when this is not necessarily the case. Parents of children with CP are encouraged to follow available trials as they recruit subjects on the www.clinicaltrials.gov Website and to scrutinize offers of treatment outside of the United States where rigorous research protocols are not used. For an overview of the current state of stem cell research in CP, please refer to a recent publication by Jantzie, which outlines the need for detailed assessments of pre- and post-intervention of patient characteristics and the use of stringent scientific principles when assessing the resultant data.[20]

DISCLOSURE STATEMENT

The author has nothing to disclose.

REFERENCES

1. Paneth N, Hong T, Korzeniewski S. The descriptive epidemiology of cerebral palsy. Clin Perinatol 2006;33:251–67.
2. Rosenbaum P, Paneth N, Leviton A, et al. A report: the definition and classification of cerebral palsy April 2006. Dev Med Child Neurol 2007;109:8–14.
3. Rosenbaum P, Palisano RJ, Bartlett DJ, et al. Development of the gross motor function classification system for cerebral palsy. Dev Med Child Neurol 2008; 50:249–53.
4. Can Child Centre for Childhood Disability Research Institute for Applied Health Sciences, McMaster University, 1400 Main Street West, Room 408, Hamilton, ON, Canada L8S 1C7. Available at: https://canchild.ca/en/resources/42-gross-motor-function-classification-system-expanded-revised-gmfcs-e-r. Accessed November 13, 2019.
5. Novak I, Morgan C, Adde L, et al. Early, accurate diagnosis and early intervention in cerebral palsy advances in diagnosis and treatment. JAMA Pediatr 2017;171: 897–907.
6. Srivastava R, Stone B, Murphy N. Hospitalist care of the medically complex child. Pediatr Clin North Am 2005;52:1165–87.
7. Ronis S, Grossberg R, Allen R, et al. Estimating nonreimbursed costs for care coordination for children with medical complexity. Pediatrics 2019;143 [pii: e20173562].
8. Sanger T. Pathophysiology of pediatric movement disorders. J Child Neurol 2003; 18:S9–24.

9. Sanger T, Delgado M, Gaebler-Spira D, et al, Task Force on Childhood Motor Disorders. Classification and definition of disorders causing hypertonia in childhood. Pediatrics 2003;111:e89–97.

10. Rice J, Skuza P, Baker F, et al. Identification and measurement of dystonia in cerebral palsy. Dev Med Child Neurol 2017;59:1249–55.

11. Carrm L, Coghill J. Mimics of cerebral palsy. Paediatr Child Health 2016;26: 387–94.

12. MacLennan A, Lewis S, Moreno-De-Luca A, et al. Genetic causation should not change the clinical diagnosis of cerebral palsy. J Child Neurol 2019;34:472–6.

13. Ostojic K, Paget SP, Morrow AM, et al. Management of pain in children and adolescents with cerebral palsy: a systematic review. Dev Med Child Neurol 2019; 61:315–21.

14. Pruitt D, Tsai T. Common medical comorbidities associated with cerebral palsy. Phys Med Rehabil Clin N Am 2009;20:453–67.

15. McLaughlin M, Walker W. Cerebral palsy – critical elements of care. Seattle (WA): The Center for Children with Special Needs Seattle Children's Hospital; 2011.

16. Available at: www.aacpdm.org/publications/care-pathways. Accessed November 13, 2019.

17. Chambers H. Selective percutaneous muscle lengthening in cerebral palsy: when there is little or no evidence. Dev Med Child Neurol 2018;60:328.

18. Canty M, Breitbart S, Siegel L, et al. The role of social media in selective dorsal rhizotomy for children: information sharing and social support. Childs Nerv Syst 2019;35(11):2179–85.

19. Novak I. Evidence-based diagnosis, health care, and rehabilitation for children with cerebral palsy. J Child Neurol 2014;8:1141–56.

20. Jantzie L, Scafidi J, Robinson S, et al. Stem cells and cell-based therapies for cerebral palsy: a call for rigor. Pediatr Res 2018;83:345–55.

APPENDIX
Box A1. National Websites with patient/parent/caregiver/provider resources

American Academy of Cerebral Palsy and Developmental Medicine	www.aacpdm.org Includes access to Care Pathways
CP Now	www.cpnowfoundation.org Includes access to The Cerebral Palsy Toolkit for Patients/Families
CP Foundation	www.yourcpf.org Reaching for the Stars is now merged with CP Foundation
My Cerebral Palsy (CP Research Network)	www.mycerebralpalsy.org A resource for individuals with CP, parents, and caregivers—to participate in research and in discussions about research priorities in CP with clinicians and other community members.

(*continued on next page*)

(continued)	
National Institute of Neurologic Disorders and Stroke	https://www.ninds.nih.gov/Disorders/All-Disorders/Cerebral-Palsy-Information-Page
Centers for Disease Control and Prevention (CDC)	www.cdc.org → Enter Cerebral Palsy https://www.cdc.gov/ncbddd/actearly/parents/states.html Information on ECI programs https://www.cdc.gov/ncbddd/actearly/milestones Resource on developmental milestones
Easter Seals and UCP which are national organizations have local affiliates	www.easterseals.org www.ucp.org
American Speech-Language-Hearing Association	https://www.asha.org Information on augmentative communication devices/evidence based literature regarding assessment and treatment of dysphagia and language impairments in CP https://www.asha.org/SLP/schools/Resources-for-school-based-SLPs/ Information geared toward SLP clinician but helpful to understand services provided to patients
Bridging Apps	www.bridgingapp.org Program launched by Easter Seals Houston as resource for families/providers on Apps for children and adults with disabilities Includes whether APP is free or at cost and with review of target audience and whether app serves to address educational and/or therapeutic goals
HUD	https://www.hud.gov/program_offices/fair_housing_equal_opp/disabilities/sect504faq Information on housing rights for individuals with disabilities
Individuals with Disabilities Education Act	https://sites.ed.gov/idea
Nemours Kids Health	https://kidshealth.org/en/parents/cerebral-palsy Condition Fact Sheets for Parents and Children/Adolescents
Stem Cell Resources	http://uclaccp.org/wp-content/uploads/Stem-cell-factsheet_Michael-Fehlings.pdf http://www.closerlookatstemcells.org/ http://clinicaltrials.gov/ct2/results?term=cerebral+palsy+AND+stem+cells
Inclusive Fitness Coalition	http://incfit.org/

Box A2. State/local Website resources with links to fact sheets/general resources (not limited to geographic area)

Disability Rights Texas	https://www.disabilityrightstx.org/en/what-we-do/service-priorities/ Contains links to resources on housing, community living, education, transportation, and health care
TexasYouth2Adult	https://www.texasyouth2adult.com Transition resource with links built by EasterSeals Greater Houston funded by Health and Human Services Grant
Baylor College of Medicine and Texas Children's Hospital	https://www.texaschildrens.org/health-professionals/conferences/20th-annual-chronic-illness-and-disability-conference-transition-pediatric-adult-based-care National conference held yearly with broadcast option on transition
Advocates for Children of New York	https://www.advocatesforchildren.org/sites/default/files/library/assistive_technology_guide.pdf?pt=1 Assistive Technology Guide for parents with explanations for navigating school evaluations and links to natlonal resources
Texas Parent to Parent	https://www.txp2p.org Parent peer support organization that also educates professionals

The Expanding Role of Genetics in Cerebral Palsy

Lisa T. Emrick, MD[a,b,*], Shannon M. DiCarlo, MD[c,1]

KEYWORDS

- Cerebral palsy • Genetics • Exome sequencing

KEY POINTS

- Cerebral palsy is a descriptive term for patients with nonprogressive motor impairments, typically thought to be associated with specific brain imaging abnormalities but now often inclusive of patients with nonprogressive genetic disorders.
- Patients with atypical presentations of cerebral palsy (normal head imaging, progressive course, family history of similar symptoms) should be considered for further genetic work-up.
- Genetic evaluation should be pursued in a stepwise fashion in order to maximize diagnostic yield with an emphasis on treatable disorders and to minimize costs.
- A genetic diagnosis may provide specific treatments for patients and reoccurrence risks to families.

INTRODUCTION

Cerebral palsy is a clinical diagnosis of a nonprogressive developmental disorder of motor impairment.[1] It was previously thought to be related to brain injury or a developmental brain malformation but the scope of the diagnosis of cerebral palsy has been broadening significantly in recent years to include patients with genetic disorders. The advent of novel genetic testing has been able to give patients who previously had a vague diagnosis of presumed or so-called MRI-negative cerebral palsy a more specific cause.

Funding: Dr Emrick received some funding as a part of the Undiagnosed Diseases Network, NIH Common Fund, through the Office of Strategic Coordination in the Office of the NIH Director under award number U01HG007709.

[a] Division of Neurology and Departmental Neurosciences, Department Pediatrics, Baylor College of Medicine, Houston, TX, USA; [b] Department of Human and Molecular Genetics, Baylor College of Medicine, Houston, TX, USA; [c] Division of Neurology and Departmental Neurosciences, Department Pediatrics, Cerebral Palsy Clinic, Baylor College of Medicine, Houston, TX, USA
[1] Present address: 15400 Southwest Freeway Suite 200, Sugarland, TX 77478.
* Corresponding author. 6701 Fannin Street, Suite 1250, Houston, TX 77030.
E-mail address: ltemrick@texaschildrens.org
Twitter: Lemrick444 (L.T.E.)

Phys Med Rehabil Clin N Am 31 (2020) 15–24
https://doi.org/10.1016/j.pmr.2019.09.006
1047-9651/20/© 2019 Elsevier Inc. All rights reserved.

There is more attention on genetic causes for cerebral palsy, and previous articles quote a range from 30%[2] to approximately between 70% and 80% of cerebral palsy attributed to perinatal causes are secondary to a genetic cause.[3] Previous literature focused on cerebral palsy masqueraders[4] and there has been an expansion as well as overlap of phenotypes of conditions with the discovery of new genes. At the time of writing, there are more than 800 genes in the Online Mendelian Inheritance in Man (OMIM) database available online at https://www.omim.org associated with cerebral palsy, representing more than 900 clinical conditions.

This article helps clinicians to determine what patients would benefit from a more thorough genetic/metabolic evaluation and helps to delineate an approach for the work-up, with an emphasis on newer technologies and the evolving fields of fetal medicine and genetics. It is not meant to be an exhaustive list of genes and conditions related to cerebral palsy but provides guidance to providers to assist in clarifying a cause for some patients' symptoms.

CEREBRAL PALSY
A Brief Definition

Cerebral palsy is a phenotypic description that includes any patient who has a nonprogressive but evolving motor impairment. The motor impairment was previously thought to be secondary to a lesion or anomaly in the brain that occurs early in development but now includes developmental brain disorders that appear structurally normal on neuroimaging. Although the disorder itself is not progressive, the clinical expression may change over time as the brain matures. Patients with cerebral palsy sometimes have associated symptoms including but not limited to disturbances in sensation, cognition, communication, perception, or behavior, and possibly including a seizure disorder.[5]

Common Risk Factors

Risk factors that predispose individuals to cerebral palsy are often divided into groups based on timing: preconception (maternal), prenatal, perinatal, and postnatal (**Table 1**).

Table 1
Risk factors for cerebral palsy

Maternal	Prenatal	Perinatal	Postnatal
• Epilepsy	• Placental abnormalities	• Prolonged delivery	• Stroke
• Thyroid disease	• Poor fetal growth	• Traumatic delivery	• Abusive head trauma
• Advanced maternal age	• Cardiac anomalies	• Breech presentation	• Meningitis
• Low socioeconomic status	• Maternal disease during pregnancy (eg, diabetes, thyroid disease, epilepsy)	• Meconium	
• Smoking	• Poor prenatal care	• Fetal hypoxia	
• Intellectual disability	• High or low amniotic fluid level	• Low APGAR scores	
• History of premature delivery	• Preeclampsia	• Seizures	
• History of multiple miscarriages	• TORCH infections	• Infection	
	• Chorioamnionitis	• Low blood sugar	
	• Twin gestation	• Jaundice	

Abbreviations: APGAR, appearance, pulse, grimace, activity, and respiration; TORCH, toxoplasmosis, other (syphilis, varicella-zoster, parvovirus B_{19}), rubella, cytomegalovirus, and herpes.
From DiCarlo S, Schwabe A. Cerebral palsy and static encephalopathies. In: Kline MW, editor. Rudolph's pediatrics. 23rd edition. New York: McGraw-Hill; 2018. p. 2672–5; with permission.

If the damage to the brain occurs after age 3 years, an alternate diagnosis is given because the spectrum of symptoms can be different when changes occur in a more developed brain.

Typical Work-up

In patients who present with a clinical picture concerning for a diagnosis of cerebral palsy, a thorough history and physical is first performed. Special attention needs to be paid to prenatal and birth history, timing of onset of symptoms, and any history of developmental plateaus or regressions. Prenatal medicine is evolving and detection of central nervous system abnormalities with the development of more sensitive fetal ultrasonography and fetal MRI is increasing as well as prenatal genetic testing.[6,7]

A family history is also important to help assess the risk of an inherited genetic condition. If possible, obtaining a 3-generation pedigree is recommended, especially if considering sending broad genetic tests such as exome or genome sequencing in order to provide the family with the most informative test results. **Table 2** provides questions suggested to ask when obtaining a family history. Genetic counselors are key members of the multidisciplinary team to help obtain thorough histories and pedigrees as well as to provide families with both pretest and posttest counseling of genetic tests.

The physical examination should include a particular focus on the neurologic and musculoskeletal components of the examination. The physical examination should also include the presence or absence of dysmorphic features that could indicate syndromic causes for patients to have abnormal tone.

If the history and examination indicate a patient with a central cause for the symptoms, imaging studies are then performed (if not done already). Some patients have imaging performed before arriving in clinic and this does not need to be repeated if it shows findings in congruence with the patient's symptoms and history. The preferred study, if one has not been done, is MRI brain without contrast, although this often requires sedation.

Once history, examination, and imaging are performed, if findings are consistent with the clinical picture, no further work-up is indicated to establish a diagnosis of cerebral palsy. The type of cerebral palsy is then classified (eg, quadriplegic, hemiplegic, diplegic, ataxic), which helps to more easily communicate the patient's diagnosis to other providers. Associated conditions are then screened for (eg, developmental delay/intellectual disability, ophthalmologic/hearing impairments, speech/language delay, feeding/swallowing dysfunction, and/or clinical events concerning for seizures) and evaluation for those conditions is performed as indicated.

Why Consider Genetic Studies?

Patients with normal MRI or other red flags listed may need further genetic work-up (**Box 1**). Patients with abnormal MRI with evidence of a developmental malformation should be evaluated for a genetic or acquired cause of a migrational abnormality. Acquired causes for migrational anomalies can include TORCH (toxoplasmosis, other [syphilis, varicella-zoster, parvovirus B_{19}], rubella, cytomegalovirus, and herpes) infections and in utero ischemia. MRI abnormalities that are found without a typical history (eg, a completely normal pregnancy and birth with findings of hypoxia on MRI) should also have further studies performed.

The main focus of this article is genetic causes that mimic cerebral palsy. However, there is an emerging area in discussing the utility of genetic testing in patients with risk factors for cerebral palsy, such as prematurity, migrational anomalies, or hypoxia.[2] Genetic testing is indicated if there is the presence of other risk factors such as a

Table 2
Relevant questions in obtaining a family history

Question	Genetic Testing Implications	Genetic Test
Is there a family history of similar motor delay?	Autosomal dominant conditions such as hereditary spastic paraparesis, dopa-responsive dystonia	Focused testing based on family history
Is there a family history of other neurodevelopmental disorders?	Neurodevelopmental condition with phenotypic heterogeneity	Focused testing based on family history
Is there a possibility of shared ancestry between parents?	Consanguinity increases risk for at least 1 if not more than 1 autosomal recessive condition	SNP-based chromosomal microarrays can detect chromosomal regions of loss of homozygosity Prefer broad sequencing testing such as whole-exome or whole-genome sequencing based on risk for multiple recessive disorders
If there is a family history of multiple miscarriages?	May be an increased risk for a chromosomal anomaly that may be secondary to an unbalanced translocation in patient	Chromosomal testing: chromosomal microarray to detect microdeletions or duplications plus karyotype to check for a translocation Karyotype in parents to detect balanced translocations
Is there a family history of other possible conditions, such as early cancer, stroke, or cardiac conditions?	Possibility of detecting other genetic conditions that may be treatable or medically actionable for the patient Decrease the chance of unsuspected incidental findings if sending exome or genome sequencing	Recommend sending exome or genome sequencing for the most complete genetic testing for the patient based on motor phenotype and family history of other possible dominantly inherited condition

Abbreviation: SNP, single nucleotide polymorphism.

suspicious family history for other affected family members, MRI findings inconsistent with the patient's clinical presentation, or the presence of other congenital anomalies.[2]

Making a genetic diagnosis can be helpful in many ways, including possible treatment options, discussing inheritance possibilities, and closure for the family. Treatment options can include specific treatment, such as in dopa-responsive dystonia or restricted diet and ammonia scavenging agents for arginase deficiency. There may be more specific treatments, such as enzyme replacement or gene therapy, for some of these conditions, such as spinal muscular atrophy. A genetic diagnosis can aid in guiding prognosis in conditions that were previously thought to be static but may be progressive; for example, a primary mitochondrial disorder or a disorder of brain iron accumulation.

Inheritance is often overlooked by nongenetic providers, but having a genetic diagnosis can help with family planning. If the patient has a genetic condition with an

---

Box 1
When to look further: red flags

- Normal MRI findings
- Imaging abnormalities isolated to the globus pallidus
- Severe symptoms in the absence of a history of perinatal injury
- Family history pattern of disease inheritance, or consanguinity
- Neurodevelopmental regression, or progressively worsening symptoms
- Isolated muscular hypotonia
- Isolated ataxia
- Rigidity (as opposed to spasticity) on physician examination
- Paraplegia

From Lee RW, Poretti A, Cohen JS, et al. A diagnostic approach for cerebral palsy in the genomic era. Neuromolecular Med. 2014;16(4):821–44; with permission.

---

autosomal recessive inheritance, there is a 1:4 chance of reoccurrence. If the genetic pathogenic variant (previously referred to as mutation) is known, then parents can consider preimplantation genetic diagnosis (PGD) versus postconception perinatal amniocentesis to test for the familial variants. PGD is a method of in vitro fertilization with selection of embryos without the known familial variant for implantation.[8] A de novo variant (not detected in either parent's blood) has a very low risk of reoccurrence if it occurred randomly in the egg or sperm before conception. There is a slight reoccurrence risk if that pathogenic variant occurs in multiple eggs or sperm secondary to germline mosaicism. It is difficult to define the reoccurrence risk because it depends on how many gametes have the pathogenic variant. The risk can range between 1% and 30% for de novo variants secondary to the possibility of germline mosaicism. It is one of the evolving areas in prenatal genetics. Parents of affected children with a known genetic pathogenic variant can still choose to do prenatal genetic diagnosis for future pregnancies, even if the variant was de novo. However, PGD can be expensive and may not be covered by insurance. Providers can refer parents of children with a suspected or confirmed genetic condition for prenatal genetic counseling for preconception options for family planning.

GENETIC TESTING OVERVIEW
Common Genetic Studies

Variations in the genetic code can lead to disruptions in the functions of the gene. Variations can occur either on a chromosomal level, such as with either microdeletions or microduplications on the chromosome, also known as copy number variants (CNVs), single nucleotide variants (SNVs), or repeat expansions. **Table 3** lists various types of genetic tests with the pros and cons/limitations for detecting these variants.

Microdeletions or microduplications have been reported in patients with diagnoses of cerebral palsy. Previous studies have reported between 10% and 12% detection rate of likely pathogenic CNV in patients with cerebral palsy.[2] The genes included in these CNVs include *KANK1*, *WDR45*, *HSPA4*, and *SPAST*.[2]

Variations can also occur secondary to single DNA nucleotide variants (SNV) that can be detected with DNA sequencing methods, such as Sanger sequencing or next-generation sequencing. Variants are classified as benign, likely benign,

Table 3
Genetic testing options

Genetic Test	Indications	Pros	Cons/Limitations
Karyotype	Specific dysmorphic features History of multiple miscarriages in mother	Trisomies including mosaicism Large chromosomal deletions Balanced chromosomal rearrangement, ring chromosomes	Does not detect microdeletions or microduplications
Chromosome microarray	Dysmorphic features Multiple congenital anomalies Associated developmental delay Nonspecific phenotype	Microdeletions and Microduplications SNP arrays: detect areas of homozygosity and uniparental disomy	Does not detect small deletions, duplications or insertions Does not detect balanced rearrangements or ring chromosomes if balanced, variants of unknown significance
Gene panel/single gene	Specific phenotypes	Better coverage than WES, may be able to detect mosaicism	Limited number of genes
WES	Nonspecific phenotype; specific phenotype but possibility of gene discovery	Broad coverage of genes Medically actionable findings	Variants of unknown significance, incidental findings, does not detect CNVs or repeat expansions
WGS	Nonspecific phenotype; specific phenotype but possibility of gene discovery	Detect single base variant (SNV), microdeletion and duplication, repeat expansions	Insurance coverage Variants of unknown significance, incidental findings
mtDNA	mtDNA-specific conditions	Specific to mtDNA genome	Heteroplasmic difference in blood and other tissues, variants of unknown significance
Repeat Expansion Panels: ataxia panel	Specific disorder	No variants of unknown significance	Limited number of genes if panel or single-gene testing

Abbreviations: mtDNA, mitochondrial DNA; WES, whole-exome sequencing; WGS, whole-genome sequencing.

pathogenic, likely pathogenic, or of unknown significance. The term variants with the qualifying statements ranging from benign to pathogenic replaced the previous terms such as mutations, polymorphisms, and benign variants or mutations secondary to some confusion around the terms and what was benign versus pathogenic.[9] Next-generation sequencing may be used in DNA panels with a specific phenotype, such as neuronal brain iron accumulation disorders. DNA panels can be helpful for specific phenotypes caused by only a few known genes but has lower detection rates in less specific phenotypes or in conditions with recent gene discovery, such as hereditary spastic paraplegia. Whole-exome sequencing (WES) or whole-genome sequencing (WGS) is recommended for testing in patient with less specific phenotypes, such as hypotonia, or if testing has a low yield from a gene panels such as hereditary spastic paraplegia.[10]

WES is DNA sequencing of the part of the genome that encodes for genes, the exons, and a small portion of the intronic sequences. It covers only about 1% of the genome. WES became clinically available in 2011 and since that time the number of genes associated with a known mendelian disorder has increased from approximately 2000 to 4000 at the end of 2018 and is still increasing. In addition to new genes being discovered, researchers also now see about 4% to 5% of patients undergoing WES who have more than 1 diagnosis,[11] and autosomal recessive conditions may arise from a pathogenic variant in 1 allele and a deletion in the other allele.[12,13] The analysis of WES results also found that there was a higher rate of de novo autosomal dominant conditions that can be detected better when using a trio-based format of sequencing the patient (the proband) and both parents to search for a de novo variant that does not exist in either parent.[13] The detection rate for making a genetic diagnosis is improving with better sequencing methods, more robust genetic bioinformatic programs to analyze the data, and more genes being discovered. However, the detection rates range between 25% and 40%. Genetic testing may show variants of unknown significance that can be difficult to prove to be pathogenic secondary to no functional testing such as a metabolic marker or in vitro assay. Providers can request reanalysis of a patient's previous WES over time or if the patient's symptoms or family history has changed. A reanalysis may lead to a diagnosis if a new gene was discovered since the initial or previous testing or if a variant of unknown significance was reclassified as pathogenic. Other reasons for the lower detection rate include pathogenic variants in noncoding regions, repeat expansions, or small deletions or duplications that may be present but were not detected on the previous testing platforms. It is hoped that the latest platform, WGS will improve the current detection rate. WGS is DNA-based sequencing of both the intronic and exonic sequences of the genome but is not currently at 100% coverage of the genome. WGS is able to detect DNA sequencing variants as well as CNVs and repeat expansions. It is becoming more clinically available by some commercial laboratories in 2019 but is expensive. The costs of testing will decrease over time with the development of newer, faster technologies. Bioinformatic tools to analyze the data will most likely also develop in the coming years to assist with interpreting and storing the data.[14]

Common Metabolic Studies

Inborn errors of metabolism can also mimic all types of cerebral palsy; for example, congenital disorders of glycosylation can present with hypotonia, dopa-responsive dystonias and arginase deficiency can present with spasticity, disorders of hyperhomocysteinuria can present with hemiplegia, and glutaric aciduria or mitochondrial dysfunction can present with dyskinesia. Leach and colleagues[15] provide a comprehensive review of treatable inborn errors of metabolism that can mimic cerebral palsy. The list of treatable disorders is increasing with newer techniques. Many of the disorders can be detected with either screening metabolic tests or, for some, more specific single tests of enzyme function. **Table 4** lists the common screening metabolic tests and disorders associated with specific types of cerebral palsy.

Initial metabolic tests usually include plasma amino acids, acylcarnitine profile, and urine organic acids. Plasma amino acids detect aminoacidurias, urea cycle disorders,

Table 4
Metabolic testing options for cerebral palsy

Cerebral Palsy Type	Metabolic Condition	Metabolic Tests
Spastic diplegia	Arginase deficiency Dopa-responsive dystonia L2 hydroxyglutaric aciduria	Plasma amino acids CSF neurotransmitters Urine organic acids
Spastic quadriplegia	Sulfite oxidase deficiency or molybdenum cofactor deficiency	Urine sulfocysteine, uric acid
	Homocysteinuria, disorders of cobalamin metabolism	Plasma amino acids, homocysteine and acylcarnitine profile, urine organic acids
Extrapyramidal	Glutaric aciduria type 1	Urine organic acids and acylglycines; plasma acylcarnitine profile
	Mitochondrial disorders	Plasma and CSF lactate, plasma and CSF amino acids (alanine), plasma acylcarnitine profile, urine organic acids
Hypotonic	Congenital disorders of glycosylation N and O linked	Serum carbohydrate transferrin include N-glycan and O-glycan analysis
	Aromatic amino decarboxylase deficiency	CNS neurotransmitters

Abbreviations: CNS, central nervous system; CSF, cerebrospinal fluid.

and some organic acidurias (argininemia, maple syrup urine disease). Acylcarnitine profile is a blood test for fatty acid oxidation disorders (small to large, not very long fatty acids; separate test for X-linked adrenoleukodystrophy and other peroxisomal disorders). The acylcarnitine profile can also assist in diagnosing aminoacidurias and organic aciduria disorders with the assistance of urine organic acid tests. Many of the disorders detected with these initial metabolic screening tests are now detected in the United States as a part of state newborn screening tests.[16] However, newborn screening tests vary by state and have been updated through the years. Therefore, what children have been screened for depends on where they were born and the year they were born.

Additional metabolic testing may be indicated depending on the patient's clinical presentation. Cerebrospinal fluid (CSF) studies can be helpful alone or with comparison of blood samples obtained around the same time to compare ratios for low levels in the CSF.

CSF amino acids and glucose compared with plasma amino acids and glucose tests are indicated if there is the presence of seizures. CSF neurotransmitters are useful if a movement disorder is present with brain MRI that is not consistent with the movements.

MANAGEMENT STRATEGIES

There are different approaches for sending genetic testing in patients with a diagnosis of cerebral palsy. If the patient's clinical history, including family history and neuroimaging, has a specific phenotype, then start with targeted testing based on that phenotype. If the features are nonspecific but there are dysmorphic features or other congenital anomalies or multiple miscarriages in the mother, then a chromosome microarray is a good test to send. If there is a history of developmental regression, then metabolic testing and an urgent referral to a specialist is recommended. Metabolic testing can also assist in characterizing a patient's phenotype and assist with more specific testing when indicated.

If the patient's phenotype is nonspecific, such as hypotonia, then consider sending a broad test such as WES if spinal muscular atrophy, myotonic dystrophy, and chromosomal abnormalities have been ruled out based on clinical history or negative testing. There are gene panels for many specific phenotypes, such as ataxia, central nervous system migrational disorders, neuromuscular disorders, and treatable disorders. There is a Web site called the Genetic Testing Registry (www.ncbi.nlm.nih.gov/gtr), which may be helpful in choosing a panel or a laboratory test to select for genetic testing. The yield of genetic testing is likely to continue to improve with advances in technology such as genomic sequencing and most likely other mechanisms such as mosaic, imprinting, or other multifactorial etiologies that have yet to be discovered. However, functional assays to assist in determining whether a variant is benign or pathogenic continue to lag behind the sequencing technology. One goal for genetic testing in the future will be to have better methods to classify genetic variants as either pathogenic or benign and to decrease the number of variants of unknown significance (VUS).

SUMMARY

Cerebral palsy was once thought to be related to acquired brain injury, but the scope of the diagnosis of cerebral palsy has been broadening significantly in recent years to include patients with genetic disorders. There are more than 800 genetic conditions in the OMIM mendelian genetic database that include cerebral palsy as a part of the phenotype. This number is expected to increase further with the improved methods for expanding the knowledge of the cause of cerebral palsy with growth of fetal medicine and genetics. At present the focus is on genetic conditions that mimic cerebral palsy motor phenotypes; however, there is ongoing work to assist with possibly identifying susceptibility genes for acquired types of cerebral palsy in the future.

DISCLOSURE

The author was a paid consultant for PTC Therapeutics regarding a rare disorder, AADC deficiency.

REFERENCES

1. Bax M, Goldstein M, Rosenbaum P, et al. Proposed definition and classification of cerebral palsy, April 2005. Dev Med Child Neurol 2005;47(8):571–6.
2. Fahey MC, Maclennan AH, Kretzschmar D, et al. The genetic basis of cerebral palsy. Dev Med Child Neurol 2017;59(5):462–9.
3. Moreno-De-Luca A, Ledbetter DH, Martin CL. Genetic [corrected] insights into the causes and classification of [corrected] cerebral palsies. Lancet Neurol 2012;11(3):283–92.
4. Lee RW, Poretti A, Cohen JS, et al. A diagnostic approach for cerebral palsy in the genomic era. Neuromolecular Med 2014;16(4):821–44.
5. Rosenbaum P, Paneth N, Leviton A, et al. A report: the definition and classification of cerebral palsy April 2006. Dev Med Child Neurol Suppl 2007;109:8–14.
6. Scher MS. Peripartum consultations expand the role of the fetal/neonatal neurologist. Pediatr Neurol 2012;47(6):411–8.

7. MacLennan AH, Thompson SC, Gecz J. Cerebral palsy: causes, pathways, and the role of genetic variants. Am J Obstet Gynecol 2015;213(6):779–88.
8. Basille C, Frydman R, El Aly A, et al. Preimplantation genetic diagnosis: state of the art. Eur J Obstet Gynecol Reprod Biol 2009;145(1):9–13.
9. Richards S, Aziz N, Bale S, et al. Standards and guidelines for the interpretation of sequence variants: a joint consensus recommendation of the American College of Medical Genetics and Genomics and the Association for Molecular Pathology. Genet Med 2015;17(5):405–24.
10. Kim A, Kumar KR, Davis RL, et al. Increased diagnostic yield of spastic paraplegia with or without cerebellar ataxia through whole-genome sequencing. Cerebellum 2019;18(4):781–90.
11. Posey JE, Harel T, Liu P, et al. Resolution of disease phenotypes resulting from multilocus genomic variation. N Engl J Med 2017;376(1):21–31.
12. Yang Y, Muzny DM, Reid JG, et al. Clinical whole-exome sequencing for the diagnosis of mendelian disorders. N Engl J Med 2013;369(16):1502–11.
13. Yang Y, Muzny DM, Xia F, et al. Molecular findings among patients referred for clinical whole-exome sequencing. JAMA 2014;312(18):1870–9.
14. Biesecker LG, Green RC. Diagnostic clinical genome and exome sequencing. N Engl J Med 2014;371(12):1170.
15. Leach EL, Shevell M, Bowden K, et al. Treatable inborn errors of metabolism presenting as cerebral palsy mimics: systematic literature review. Orphanet J Rare Dis 2014;9:197.
16. American College of Medical Genetics Newborn Screening Expert Group. Newborn screening: toward a uniform screening panel and system–executive summary. Pediatrics 2006;117(5 Pt 2):S296–307.

Optimizing Nutrition and Bone Health in Children with Cerebral Palsy

Anna O. Jesus, MD[a], Richard D. Stevenson, MD[b],*

KEYWORDS

- Cerebral palsy • Nutrition • Growth • Bone health • Surgery

KEY POINTS

- Growth and nutritional status are challenging to assess in children with CP, yet the consequences of poor growth and malnutrition are vast, ranging from decreased bone density and muscle mass to decreased participation in everyday activities.
- Malnutrition, exposure to certain medications, and intrinsic differences in muscle mass, tone, and function increase a child with CP's risk of compromised bone health.
- Optimizing bone health often focuses on prevention rather than treatment of reduced bone mineral density.
- Good nutritional care in the period leading up to and surrounding major surgery is associated with improved wound healing, muscle strength, and coughing strength, as well as decreased length of stay and mortality.

INTRODUCTION

Children with cerebral palsy (CP) are at risk of growth and nutrition disorders, which tend to become more clinically important with increasing severity of motor impairments.[1,2] Children with CP can present with challenges to nutritional intake, including swallowing disorders and constipation, difficulties communicating hunger and satiety, fatigue, and risk of aspiration, and are therefore at risk of malnutrition.[3] Consequences of malnutrition may include:

- Decreased bone density, and therefore increased fracture risk
- Decreased muscle mass, leading to weakness, increased risk of aspiration, and decreased functional status

Disclosure Statement: The authors have nothing to disclose.
[a] University of Virginia, UVA Neurodevelopmental and Behavioral Pediatrics, Stacey Hall, PO Box 800828, Charlottesville, VA 22908, USA; [b] Division of Neurodevelopmental and Behavioral Pediatrics, University of Virginia School of Medicine, University of Virginia, UVA Neurodevelopmental and Behavioral Pediatrics, Stacey Hall, PO Box 800828, Charlottesville, VA 22908, USA
* Corresponding author.
E-mail address: rds8z@hscmail.mcc.virginia.edu

Phys Med Rehabil Clin N Am 31 (2020) 25–37
https://doi.org/10.1016/j.pmr.2019.08.001
1047-9651/20/© 2019 Elsevier Inc. All rights reserved.

- Decreased quality of life, including increased missed days of school and work, decreased ability to play and participate in therapies
- Decreased neurodevelopmental potential, including intellectual quotient, school achievement, behavior, and attention
- Decreased immune function, with increased infection risk and prolonged wound healing
- Increased health care costs

Growth in childhood is often used as a proxy for health and well-being. Yet even with the appropriate environment and regular medical attention, children with CP grow more slowly than children without chronic health conditions.[4] Furthermore, reliable measurements of growth (typically height and weight) are difficult to obtain in children with CP owing to fixed joint contractures, scoliosis, involuntary muscle spasms, or poor cooperation because of cognitive defects,[5,6] creating further challenges to following growth as a reflection of nutrition and health.

This article discusses how to appropriately assess growth and nutrition in children with CP, why addressing inadequate growth and nutrition is critical to health and well-being, methods of optimizing nutrition and bone health, and additional considerations when preparing for and recovering from surgery.

ASSESSMENT OF GROWTH AND NUTRITION IN CHILDREN WITH CEREBRAL PALSY

Part of routine health care maintenance for every child is surveillance of growth and nutritional status. Although the same is true for children with CP, other considerations must be taken into account when interpreting growth and nutrition. Height and weight remain useful tools for establishing growth when possible. However, they are less helpful in determining percent body fat, particularly in more severely impaired children. Triceps and subscapular skinfold thickness are validated indicators for estimating body fat. Standard techniques are well established in children with disabilities, and some evidence suggests that an essential element for the assessment of nutritional status in children with CP is triceps skinfold thickness.[7]

Once reliable anthropometric measurements are obtained, assessing nutritional status is not as straightforward as it is with children without chronic medical conditions. Standard growth curves for height or length, weight, head circumference, and body mass index (weight in kilograms/height in meters squared) have been developed by the Centers for Disease Control and Prevention (CDC) and the World Health Organization (WHO). Although differences exist between the growth charts—the CDC compiled cross-sectional data from only the United States, and the WHO included mixed longitudinal data from multiple countries—both are based on studies of typically active children and, therefore, demonstrate how an otherwise healthy child did grow (CDC) or should grow (WHO).[8]

However, children with CP do not grow "normally," even with optimal nutritional intake and environmental components, and the growth differences correlate with functional severity. The exact mechanistic causes of growth differences are not understood but likely include differences in nutrition, hormones, movement-induced growth, genetics (at least in some cases), and other unknown factors. CP-specific growth charts are available based on the severity of gross motor impairment.[9] Higher levels of impairment correlate with poorer growth. Although these CP-specific growth charts are useful guides for monitoring growth (particularly weight and weight gain), these charts portray how a large clinical sample of children with CP *has* grown and not necessarily what is optimal growth with appropriate nutrition.[10,11]

In addition to assessing adequate growth using anthropometric measurements during a point in time, it is critical to monitor weight gain trends over time in the context of energy intake in relation to needs. If a child is growing along his/her expected curve, it is likely appropriate growth.[12] Several equations are available to help estimate energy needs depending on age, sex, and ambulatory status.[13] After a baseline estimate is determined, close follow-up of weight is required to assess whether the estimate is adequate, inadequate, or excessive.

Physical characteristics, in particular hair, skin, nails, and pubertal status, also serve as indicators of nutritional state (**Table 1**). Of note, although sexual maturation may be indicative of adequate nutritional state, a cross-sectional analysis of children with moderate to severe CP showed a complex relationship between sexual maturation and body fat, perhaps mirroring typical differences in pubertal girls and boys. For girls with CP, more advanced sexual maturation was associated with higher percent body fat. For boys with CP, however, more advanced sexual maturation was associated with less body fat.[14]

Laboratory assessment may be helpful both in gauging the presence of inadequate nutrition and, in specific situations, in determining causality (**Table 2**). Decreased albumin is often suggestive of chronic malnutrition, but it is also affected by inflammation and fluid shifts, therefore it has questionable clinical use.[16]

Combining many of these individual assessments, the Subjective Global Assessment (SGA) is a validated and reproducible technique that has been used in adults for over 30 years. It takes into consideration weight, dietary intake, gastrointestinal symptoms, functional status, and physical examination. In the adult context, SGA can predict nutrition-associated complications (ie, infections, use of antibiotics, length of stay) better than serum albumin, transferrin, delayed cutaneous hypersensitivity, the

Table 1
Physical characteristics and possible nutritional deficiencies

	Physical Examination Finding	Possible Nutritional Deficiency
Hair	Lanugo (fine, soft hair over the trunk)	Malnutrition
	Alopecia	Protein calories
Skin	Pallor	Iron
		Folate
		Cobalamin
	Lesions or fissures in the oral cavity	Vitamin B
	Pressure ulcers and poor wound healing	Protein calories
		Vitamin C
		Vitamin D
		Zinc
Nails	Beau's lines (transverse ridges or horizontal grooves)	Protein
		Zinc
		Calcium
	Koilonychia (spoon-shaped nails)	Protein
		Vitamin B9 (folic acid)
		Vitamin B12 (cobalamin)
		Iron
	Brittle, soft, thin nails	Severe calorie malnutrition
		Vitamin A
		Magnesium
		Selenium
Pubertal status	Delays	Calorie malnutrition

Table 2 Clinical concerns and laboratory assessments	
Clinical Concern	**Laboratory Assessment**
Decreased bone mineral density[15]	Vitamin D (25-OH) Alkaline phosphatase Calcium Phosphorus
Anemia	Complete blood cell count
Electrolyte disarray or renal failure	Basic metabolic panel

Prognostic Nutrition Index, creatinine-height index, triceps skinfold thickness, and various combinations of these measures.[17] Recently, the SGA has been suggested as a tool for pediatric patients with CP, and 1 validation study shows promise.[18]

IMPACT OF NUTRITIONAL STATUS ON HEALTH AND SOCIETAL PARTICIPATION

Although the consequences of malnutrition in children without disabilities have been well studied,[19] research in children with motor disabilities is less well described, with many experts believing that the effects on unaffected individuals are applicable to undernourished children with CP.[10] Furthermore, the evidence regarding some of the benefits of adequate nutrition, such as its relationship to surgical morbidity, specifically in children with CP is conflicting.[20–22]

However, poor growth and nutrition could be a contributing factor to (rather than solely a reflection of) a child's medical complexity and its subsequent encumbrance on the life of both child and caregivers. The North American Growth in Cerebral Palsy Project (NAGCPP) correlated nutritional status with health care use and societal participation in a population-based sample of children with moderate to severe CP.[23] The study found a statistically significant relationship between mid-upper arm fat area and subscapular skinfold thickness and health care use, child participation in school and usual activities, and parent participation in their usual activities. Using the negative binomial regression model, this effect was independent of GMFCS level, age, and gender. Each standard deviation decrease in mid-upper arm fat area was associated with a 28% increase in doctor visits, 31% increase in days missed from school, and a 51% increase in missed activities for the family throughout the preceding 4 weeks.

Four years later, NAGCPP developed CP-specific growth curves, and clustered subjects based on the Z scores on 6 measures of growth and body composition.[1] When correlated with markers of health and social participation, larger children had fewer days of health care and missed days of usual activities, although these findings were not statistically significant. When neurologic severity was taken into account, 2 of the health and participation measures (missed days at school and days of usual activities missed by family members) were statistically significant. NAGCPP helped illustrate the profound impact of poor growth on a child's life, including his/her present day-to-day life in addition the more abstract long-term consequences. There have not been more recent studies that examine this effect.

BONE HEALTH

Bone growth, evaluated by length and bone density, is an important aspect of growth in children with CP. Children with CP are at higher risk of compromised bone health, in part owing to underlying malnutrition from multiple causes—inadequate intake, intolerance to feeds, or fatigue.[24] Children with CP who feed orally typically take longer to feed and take in only a small proportion of that offered to them.[25] In an evaluation of 117 subjects with moderate to severe CP, difficulty feeding the child (as reported by the caregiver) and lower triceps skinfold scores were strong predictors of lower bone mineral density in both the distal femur and the lumbar spine.[26]

Inadequate nutrition often correlates with low levels of calcium, vitamin D, and phosphorus, which are the chief nutrients of concern for bone health. However, in the study described above, serum 25-hydroxy vitamin D levels did not correlate with bone mineral density. A previous study demonstrated that low calcium intake was a contributor to low bone mineral density, but serum calcium, alkaline phosphatase, and vitamin D levels were not found to correlate.[27]

Certain medications are thought to negatively impact bone health by blocking or altering the absorption or metabolism of nutrients or by altering the metabolic processes of the body.[24] Unfortunately, several of these medications are commonly taken by children with CP, such as anticonvulsants (particularly phenobarbital and phenytoin), proton-pump inhibitors, antidepressants, and depot medroxyprogesterone acetate.[28] Evidence on the impact of anticonvulsants on bone density has been mixed. Henderson and colleagues'[27] 1995 study on patients with CP across GMFCS levels demonstrated a correlation between anticonvulsant use and bone mineral density, but the relationship was not present once severity of CP and nutritional status were controlled. Henderson and colleagues'[26] 2002 study focusing on children with moderate to severe CP (GMFCS III-V) did demonstrate a correlation.

In addition to malnutrition and nutrient deficiency, weight-bearing status, likely in combination with the impact of muscle mass and active muscle contraction and movement, plays a role in diminished bone health in children with CP. It has been well documented in otherwise healthy children and adolescents that lack of weight bearing or immobilization results in decreased bone mineral density and, consequently, bones that are more susceptible to fracture.[29,30] Forces on the bone help regulate the modeling and remodeling of bone through osteoblast and osteoclast activity. Lack of weight-bearing results in reduced periosteal expansion. Non- and minimally ambulatory children with CP have been found to have smaller and thinner tibiae with decreased cortical bone area than children with CP who can walk.[31,32]

There is also an association between GMFCS level, independent of ambulatory status, and bone mineral density. Henderson and colleagues[26] found that bone mineral density Z scores were significantly lower in GMFCS level 5 children than in level 4 children, despite the fact that both groups were non-ambulatory. In discussion, they compared boys with Duchenne muscular dystrophy, who tend to have dramatically diminished bone mineral density in the femurs years before they become non-ambulatory. Although corticosteroid use could be a confounder, interestingly, these boys had relatively preserved bone mineral density in the lumbar spine before loss of ambulation.[33] Thus, there are likely multiple factors intrinsic to CP, such as atypical muscle tone and function, that contribute to differences in bone growth[24] independent of weight bearing per se.

With differences in bone growth and density, there is concern for fracture risk in children with CP. In a longitudinal cohort study by Stevenson and colleagues[34] of 245 patients with moderate to severe CP, 15.7% were reported to have a history of fractures at baseline. Surprisingly, although increasing GMFCS level has been shown to be a risk factor for lower bone mineral density, it was not found to be significant in this study. Based on 24 fractures in 604.5 person-years of prospective follow-up, the fracture rate was 4.0% per year. For children with a history of previous fracture, the fracture rate increased to 7.0% per year. Having a gastrostomy and a higher percent body fat also correlated with higher fracture rate, at 6.8% per year and 9.7% per year, respectively; the authors hypothesized that higher body fat could, in part, be a marker for less lean mass.

INTERVENTIONS FOR OPTIMIZING NUTRITION FOR BONE HEALTH

The main focus on preventing low bone density should be to ensure that nutrition is adequate. If there is concern for malnutrition, it is helpful to involve a dietician or a gastroenterologist to assess the causes and provide recommendations for appropriate intake, as well as a speech/language or occupational therapist to assess feeding and ensure that the child is safely and efficiently consuming an adequate diet.[13] Instituting a meal schedule (3 meals plus 2–3 snacks) that provides a child with multiple opportunities to eat nutrient-rich foods (including proteins, fruits, vegetables, whole grains, and dairy) is a crucial first step in increasing daily calorie intake. Oral nutrition supplements, such as heavy cream, whole milk, butter, cheese, peanut butter, avocado, or complete enteral nutrition formulas, which dieticians favor since they meet the basic macro- and micronutrient requirements,[35] are often necessary to increase calorie, and protein, and micronutrient intake.

Because children with CP are at increased risk for poor bone health, special attention must be given to make sure a diet is complete, with appropriate intake of calcium, phosphorus, vitamin D, zinc, and magnesium. Calcium is primarily found in dairy products, although soy, legume, and some fish are also good sources. For a child with feeding challenges, calcium and phosphorus intake should be evaluated. Additional calcium supplementation used to be common in both children and adults in an effort to improve bone mineral density. Although similar studies in children have not been replicated, several large randomized controlled trials have found an association between calcium supplements and cardiovascular events, in addition to constipation, gastrointestinal symptoms, and kidney stones,[36] making its use more limited. Vitamin D supplementation, however, is routinely recommended in children with CP. In those who are non-ambulatory, it is recommended that their serum 25-hydroxy vitamin D level is at least 30 to 40 ng/mL.[24] To achieve these levels, most children require additional supplementation of 1000 to 8000 IU units daily, particularly if sun exposure is limited.[37] In patients who are severely deficient, or if daily compliance is a concern, an alternative "stoss therapy" (from the German word *stossen*, meaning "to push") can be used. Doses of 100,000 to 600,000 units of vitamin D can be given orally as a single dose, followed by a maintenance regimen described above.[37,38] The pediatric Kidney Disease Outcomes Quality Initiative provided guidelines for safe, high-dose administration of vitamin D.[39]

ADDITIONAL INTERVENTIONS FOR IMPROVING BONE HEALTH

As previously described, weight-bearing status helps maintain bone mineral density and reduce fracture risk in children with CP. At this time, only small, uncontrolled studies report a positive effect of standing on bone density and a temporary reduction in spasticity.[40] The most recent studies support a positive impact on bone density and possibly bone length, but neither is statistically significant, suggesting that more than simply the act of applying static load to bone but rather dynamic weight bearing is required to make a difference in density.[41] Furthermore, the impact of weight bearing is mostly geared toward prevention, not treatment of bone fragility. Positioning children with complex CP in standers can be challenging and many cannot tolerate as much as an hour a day (the frequency typically associated with a positive impact on bone density). It is imperative to have a pediatric physical therapist assess the type of stander (prone, supine, sit-to-stand) or gait-trainer that would be appropriate and safe for the child to use, especially if there is already concern for decreased bone mineral density.

In addition to vitamin D supplementation, bisphosphonates can be considered in further pharmacologic management of bone fragility. Bisphosphonates increase bone mineral density by inactivating osteoclasts, which are responsible for the breakdown of existing bone cells. They are widely used in the treatment of adult osteoporosis, but their use in children is controversial due to lack of long-term safety and efficacy data.[42,43] In children, the most common side effects are related to an acute phase reaction, involving fever, bone pain, nausea, and vomiting.[24] These side effects typically respond well to non-steroidal anti-inflammatory drugs and are less severe during subsequent treatments. Hypocalcemia and hypophosphatemia can occur and serum levels of these and vitamin D must be monitored. Two serious rare side effects have been well-documented in adults but have not been seen in children: osteonecrosis of the jaw and atypical femur fractures. The incidence of the former is highest in those who have had recent invasive dental procedures, have poor oral hygiene or preexisting dental disease, or who are immunocompromised.[44] The latter is associated with long-term use, leading physicians to often limit therapy to 5 years.

Given the risks associated with long-term use in the adult literature, typically treatment is limited to a year. Studies with pamidronate demonstrate that bone mineral density typically increases during the period of treatment, and then decreases back to baseline within 2 years of discontinuation.[45,46] Despite this return, a high proportion of children remain fracture free for 5 years or more. A protocol for a Cochrane Review on the use of bisphosphonates in children with CP is currently underway.[47]

PREPARING FOR SURGERY

Children with CP who undergo surgery, particularly spinal surgery that is invasive and requires a lengthy recovery period, should have nutritional status evaluated closely. Although there is some conflicting evidence on the benefits of preoperative nutrition in children with CP and post-operative complications,[21] we know that good nutrition in children with CP improves general health,[9] decreases lengths of hospital stays,[23] improves bone health,[26] and is a powerful prognosticator of survival.[9] It is therefore advisable for children with CP who are preparing for surgery to be evaluated by a nutrition support team to determine if oral or enteral feeds can be improved.

Oral feeding plans should focus on improving the feeding process (positioning, altering viscosity, texture and sensory awareness of the food, pacing of the meal, finding appropriate utensils, and balancing fatigue with the pleasure of eating) and optimizing intake. Prediction equations for estimating energy requirements that have been validated in typically developing children do not perform well in children with CP.[48] Initial equations to estimate energy requirements have proven inaccurate.[49] A more recent study by Walker and colleagues[50] demonstrated that energy requirements decrease as ambulatory status declines and more limbs are involved, and that the best predictor of energy requirement is fat-free mass, rather than ambulatory status. Dr. Gina Rempel summarizes goals for pre-operative nutrition in the malnourished child in affiliation with the American Academy for Cerebral Palsy and Developmental Medicine (AACPDM) (**Table 3**).[51]

Sometimes these goals cannot be met by oral feeding alone, despite potential adjustments described above. Abnormalities in tone and difficulties with motor coordination in children with CP can result in persistent oral-motor dysfunction or dysphasia.

Table 3	
Nutrition rehabilitation goals for children with poor nutritional status in the pre-operative period	
Nutrients	Protein and micronutrients (including vitamin D and calcium) requirements similar to matched peers.
	If undernourished, aim for caloric intake at least 10% above current intake.
Triceps skin fold	Aim for 10–25th percentile for age.
Weight	Monitor at 2- to 4-wk intervals.
Weight gain velocity	Aim for 4–7 gm/d in children >1 y, adjusting with degree of malnutrition.
Weight for age on CP growth chart	Aim for weight >20th percentile.

From Rempel G. Optimizing nutrition for children with cerebral palsy undergoing spinal surgery. Available at: https://www.aacpdm.org/UserFiles/file/IC22-Dietz-2.pdf. Accessed January 27, 2019; with permission.

Oral-motor dysfunction may be a presenting feature of CP in early infancy, or it may develop as children age and struggle with mastery of complex voluntary and learned motor movements necessary for safe and efficient biting, chewing, and swallowing. Prognostic criteria for sufficient, safe, and efficient dietary intake, or conversely for the need of gastrostomy, have not been established. Decision-making around the need and timing for gastrostomy requires clinical judgment, and ideally a family-focused, team approach. Prolonged feeding times and insufficient intake lead to poor growth, and a gastrostomy tube may be considered to improve nutritional status sufficiently before surgery. A gastrostomy tube might also be considered if the child suffers from a large number or high severity of respiratory illnesses, or if concerns for safety and quantity of nutrition detract from pleasant mealtime interactions.[13] Placement of a gastrostomy tube does not preclude oral feeding, and families and children generally experience improved quality of life and better health after placement.[52,53]

PERI- AND POST-OPERATIVE MANAGEMENT

Providing good nutritional care is fundamental in the period surrounding major surgery, especially in the intensive care setting. No perioperative nutrition care guidelines are available, but a Care Pathway in affiliation with the AACPDM is under development. In addition to enhancing immune function, hastening wound healing, and decreasing length of stay and mortality, adequate nutrition also improves muscle strength and decreases respiratory muscle weakness, therefore improving coughing strength.[54] These differences can have an impact on aspects of immediate postoperative care such as intubation times, ability to participate in therapy and other measures designed to help minimize the risk of complications such as pneumonia, atelectasis, and bed wounds.

When creating a nutritional plan, careful attention should be made toward ensuring appropriate protein intake, which is associated with decreased 60-day mortality in the pediatric intensive care unit. Energy requirements do not increase in the postoperative period, but protein needs do.[51] Delivery of over 60% of the prescribed protein intake is associated with a lower mortality in mechanically ventilated children.[55]

Enteral nutrition should be encouraged over parental nutrition. When possible, nutrition should be provided in a way that is most physiologic. As long as there is peristalsis of the gut, trophic feeds improve the gastrointestinal environment.[56] In contrast with parental nutrition, which requires at least peripheral if not central intravenous access, enteral nutrition is not associated with increased risk of infection or increased length of stay.[56] It is also often well tolerated, even in conjunction with vasopressor use.[57] Of note, there are no clear improvements in the risks of aspiration, pneumonia, or feeding tolerance with the use of continuous instead of bolus feeds[51]; bolus feeds are more physiologic and should help promote gastric emptying and gastrointestinal motility. Care must be taken not to over feed through gastrostomy to avoid vomiting. Elevating the head of the bed during feeding can decrease the risk of ventilator-associated pneumonia. Constipation is common in this population (in the setting of opiate use following surgery, post-operative ileus, and abnormal muscle tone at baseline), and must be aggressively managed to promote feeding tolerance.

AREAS FOR DISCOVERY

As discussed, the development of SGA to screen for malnutrition is beginning to be considered in children with CP. Currently it is widely used as a valid tool for the nutritional diagnosis of hospitalized clinical and surgical adult patients. More recently, a modified version called the subjective global nutritional assessment (SGNA) was adapted for use in children, with some studies demonstrating validity and reliability in preoperative and pediatric intensive care unit patients.[58,59] Several factors from a nutrition-focused medical history and physical examination are used to generate an SGNA rating. Moving forward, a group of factors most pertinent to children with CP should be developed and validated to help classify nutritional status, and then determine if the resulting SGA/SGNA can be predictive of nutrition-associated health complications.

There are also several potential treatments for bone fragility that merit further research, including the use of exogenous growth hormone and low frequency (or whole-body) vibration. There is abundant data that growth hormone therapy leads to an increase in bone mineral density in children with growth hormone deficiency.[60,61] In 1 pilot randomized control study of 10 children with CP and osteopenia, but without known growth hormone deficiency, both linear growth and bone mineral density increased significantly in the group treated with growth hormone over 18 months.[62] Side effects were minimal, although treatment does require daily subcutaneous injection. Larger prospective studies are needed to better discern clinical significance and exclude possible confounders.

In whole-body vibration, the child sits or lies on a machine with a vibrating platform; vibrations force the muscles to contract and relax quickly. In 1 small randomized control trial, children with CP who received low-level mechanical stimulation had improved bone mineral density in the tibia after 6 months.[63] A more recent study found a paradoxic change in density of participants' femurs.[64] In the intervention group there was an increase within the distal femur metaphysis but a significant decrease in density in the femoral diaphysis. The authors hypothesized that these findings could be attributed to inaccurate assessments of bone density because of challenges performing densitometry in the distal femur of the patients in their study. No change was noted in the bone density of the lumbar spine. A 2015 systematic review concluded that there is a lack of research to conclude whether whole body vibration alters bone mineral density.[65] Particularly, given that this adjunct therapy appears safe, time-efficient, and promising in terms of building strength, decreasing spasticity, and increasing functionality, more research should be performed to evaluate its effects on bone mineral density.

SUMMARY

Growth and nutritional status has many profound effects on the lives of children with CP. Appropriate assessment of both poses several challenges and requires a multi-modal, longitudinal, and interdisciplinary approach. Optimizing nutrition is beneficial for bone health as well as peri- and post-operative morbidity and mortality. Further research should now be directed toward adjunct treatments to further promote bone health and improve perioperative outcomes in children with CP.

REFERENCES

1. Stevenson RD, Conaway M, Chumlea WC, et al. Growth and health in children with moderate-to-severe cerebral palsy. Pediatrics 2006;118:1010–8.
2. Day S, Strauss D, Vachon P, et al. Growth patterns in a population of children and adolescents with cerebral palsy. Dev Med Child Neurol 2007;49:167–71.
3. Caselli TB, Lomazi EA, Montenegro MAS, et al. Assessment of nutritional status of children and adolescents with spastic quadriplegic cerebral palsy. Arq Gastroenterol 2017;54(3):201–5.
4. Samson-Fang LJ, Stevenson RD. Linear growth velocity in children with cerebral palsy. Dev Med Child Neurol 1998;40:689–92.
5. Spender QW, Cronk CE, Charney EB, et al. Assessment of linear growth of children with cerebral palsy: use of alternative measure to height or length. Dev Med Child Neurol 1989;36:135–42.
6. Tobis JS, Saturen P, Larios G, et al. Study of growth patterns in cerebral palsy. Arch Phys Med Rehabil 1961;42:475–81.
7. Samson-Fang L, Stevenson R. Identification of malnutrition in children with cerebral palsy: poor performance of weight-for-height centiles. Dev Med Child Neurol 2000;42(3):162–8.
8. Ogden CL, Kuczmarski RJ, Flegal KM, et al. Centers for Disease Control and Prevention 2000 growth charts for the United States: improvements to the 1977 National Center for Health Statistics version. Pediatrics 2002;109:45–60.
9. Brooks J, Day S, Shavelle R, et al. Low weight, morbidity, and mortality in children with cerebral palsy: new clinical growth charts. Pediatrics 2011;128:e299–307.
10. Kuperminc MN, Stevenson RD. Growth and nutrition disorders in children with cerebral palsy. Dev Disabil Res Rev 2008;14:137–46.
11. Krick J, Murphy-Miller P, Zeger S, et al. Pattern of growth in children with cerebral palsy. J Am Diet Assoc 1996;96:680–5.
12. Kuperminc MN, Gottrand F, Samson-Fang L, et al. Nutritional management of children with cerebral palsy: a practical guide. Eur J Clin Nutr 2013;67:S21–3.
13. Bickley MC, Delaney E, Intagliata V. Feeding and nutrition. In: Glader LJ, Stevenson RD, editors. Children and youth with complex cerebral palsy: care and management. London: Mac Keith Press; 2019. p. 107–29.
14. Worley G, Houlihan C, Herman-Giddens M, et al. Secondary sexual characteristics in children with cerebral palsy and moderate to severe motor impairment: a cross-sectional survey. Pediatrics 2002;110(5):897–902.
15. Fehlings D, Switzer L, Agarwal P, et al. Informing evidence-based clinical practice guidelines for children with cerebral palsy at risk of osteoporosis: a systematic review. Dev Med Child Neurol 2012;54(2):106–16.
16. Samson-Fang L, Be KL. Assessment of growth and nutrition in children with cerebral palsy. Eur J Clin Nutr 2013;67:S5–8.
17. Baker JP, Detsky AS, Wesson DE, et al. Nutritional assessment: a comparison of clinical judgment and objective measurements. N Engl J Med 1982;306:969–72.

18. Minocha P, Sitaraman S, Choudhary A, et al. Subjective Global Nutritional Assessment: a reliable screening tool for nutritional assessment in cerebral palsy children. Indian J Pediatr 2008;85:15.

19. Stevenson RD. Nutrition and growth. In: Accardo PJ, editor. Capute & Accardo's neurodevelopmental disabilities in infancy and childhood. The spectrum of neurodevelopmental disabilities, vol 2, 3rd edition. Baltimore (MD): Brookes Publishing; 2008. p. p129–43.

20. Jevsevar DS, Karlin LI. The relationship between preoperative nutritional-status and complications after an operation for scoliosis in patients who have cerebral palsy. J Bone Joint Surg Am 1993;75(6):880–4.

21. Lipton G, Miller F, Dabney K, et al. Factors predicting postoperative complications following spinal fusions in children with cerebral palsy. J Spinal Disord 1999;12(3):197–205.

22. Weber T. A prospective analysis of factors influencing outcome after fundoplication. J Pediatr Surg 1995;30(7):1061–4.

23. Samson-Fang L, Fung E, Stallings VA, et al. Relationship of nutritional status to health and societal participation in children with cerebral palsy. J Pediatr 2002; 41(5):637–43.

24. Bachrach SJ, Kecskemethy HH. Osteoporosis and fractures. In: Glader LJ, Stevenson RD, editors. Children and youth with complex cerebral palsy: care and management. London: Mac Keith Press; 2019. p. 87–105.

25. Gisel EG, Patrick J. Identification of children with cerebral palsy unable to maintain a normal nutritional state. Lancet 1988;1(8580):283–6.

26. Henderson RC, Lark RK, Gurka MJ, et al. Bone density and metabolism in children and adolescents with moderate to severe cerebral palsy. Pediatrics 2002; 110:e5.

27. Henderson RC, Lin PP, Greene WB. Bone-mineral density in children and adolescents who have spastic cerebral palsy. J Bone Joint Surg Am 1995;77:1671–81.

28. Kecskemethy HH, Harcke HT. Assessment of bone health in children with disabilities. J Pediatr Rehabil Med 2014;7:111–24.

29. Giangregorio L, McCartney N. Bone loss and muscle atrophy in spinal cord injury: epidemiology, fracture prediction, and rehabilitation strategies. J Spinal Cord Med 2006;29(5):489–500.

30. Ceroni D, Martin X, Delhumeau C, et al. Effects of cast-mediated immobilization on bone mineral mass at various sites in adolescents with lower-extremity fracture. J Bone Joint Surg Am 2012;94A(3):208–16.

31. Binkley T, Johnson J, Vogel L, et al. Bone measurements by peripheral quantitative computed tomography (pQCT) in children with cerebral palsy. J Pediatr 2005;147(6):791–6.

32. Al Wren T, Lee DC, Kay RM, et al. Bone density and size in ambulatory children with cerebral palsy. Dev Med Child Neurol 2011;53(2):137–41.

33. Larson CM, Henderson RC. Bone mineral density and fractures in boys with Duchenne muscular dystrophy. J Pediatr Orthop 2000;20:71–4.

34. Stevenson RD, Conaway M, Barrington JW, et al. Fracture rate in children with cerebral palsy. Pediatr Rehabil 2006;9:396–403.

35. Brown B, Roehl K, Betz M. Enteral nutrition formula selection: current evidence and implication for practice. Nutr Clin Pract 2015;30(1):72–85.

36. Bolland MJ, Grey A, Reid IR. Calcium supplements and cardiovascular risk: 5 years on. Ther Adv Drug Saf 2013;4(5):199–210.

37. Hochberg Z, Bereket A, Davenport M, et al. Consensus development for the supplementation of vitamin D in childhood and adolescence. Horm Res 2002;58(1): 39–51.
38. Shah BR, Finberg L. Single-day therapy for nutritional vitamin D-deficiency rickets: a preferred method. J Pediatr 1994;125(3):487–90.
39. Lee JY, So TY, Thackray J. A review on vitamin D deficiency treatment in pediatric patients. J Pediatr Pharmacol Ther 2013;18(4):277–91.
40. Pin TW. Effectiveness of static weight-bearing exercises in children with cerebral palsy. Pediatr Phys Ther 2007;19(1):62–73.
41. Han EY, Choi JH, Kim SH, et al. The effect of weight bearing on bone mineral density and bone growth in children with cerebral palsy: a randomized controlled preliminary trial. Medicine 2017;96(10):e5896.
42. Allington N, Vivegnis D, Gerard P. Cyclic administration of pamidronate to treat osteoporosis in children with cerebral palsy or a neuromuscular disorder: a clinical study. Acta Orthop Belg 2005;71(1):91–7.
43. Boyce AM, Tosi LL, Paul SM. Bisphosphonate treatment for children with disabling conditions. PM R 2014;6(5):427–36.
44. Khan AA, Morrison A, Hanley DA, et al. Diagnosis and management of osteonecrosis of the jaw: a systematic review and international consensus. J Bone Miner Res 2015;30(1):3–23.
45. Bachrach SJ, Kecskemethy HH, Harcke H. Decreased fracture incidence after 1 year of pamidronate treatment in children with spastic quadriplegic cerebral palsy. Dev Med Child Neurol 2010;52(9):837–42.
46. Henderson RC, Lark RK, Kecskemethy HH, et al. Bisphosphonates to treat osteopenia in children with quadriplegic cerebral palsy: a randomized placebo-controlled clinical trial. J Pediatr 2002;141:644–51.
47. Zareen Z, McDonnell C, McDonald D, et al. Bisphosphonate use in children with cerebral palsy. Cochrane Database Syst Rev 2017;(8):CD012756.
48. Stallings VA, Zemel BS, Davies JC, et al. Energy expenditure of children and adolescents with severe disabilities: a cerebral palsy model. Am J Clin Nutr 1996; 64(4):627–34.
49. Rieken R, van Goudoever JB, Schierbeek H, et al. Measuring body composition and energy expenditure in children with severe neurologic impairment and intellectual disability. Am J Clin Nutr 2011;94(3):759–66.
50. Walker JL, Bell KL, Boyd RN, et al. Energy requirements in preschool-age children with cerebral palsy. Am J Clin Nutr 2012;96(6):1309–15.
51. Rempel G. Optimizing nutrition for children with cerebral palsy undergoing spinal surgery. In: AACPDM. Available at: https://www.aacpdm.org/UserFiles/file/IC22-Dietz-2.pdf. Accessed January 27, 2019.
52. Mahant S, Friedman JN, Connolly B, et al. Tube feeding and quality of life in children with severe neurological impairment. Arch Dis Child 2009;94:668–73.
53. Sleigh G, Brocklehurst P. Gastrostomy feeding in cerebral palsy: a systematic review. Arch Dis Child 2004;89:534–9.
54. Andrew M, Parr J, Sullivan P. Feeding difficulties in children with CP. Arch Dis Child Educ Pract Ed 2012;97:222–9.
55. Mehta NM, Bechard LJ, Cahill N, et al. Nutritional practices and their relationship to clinical outcomes in critically ill children—an international multicenter cohort study. Crit Care Med 2012;40:2204–11.
56. Hamilton S, McAleer D, Ariagno K, et al. A stepwise enteral nutrition algorithm for critically ill children helps achieve nutrient delivery goals. Pediatr Crit Care Med 2014;15(7):583–9.

57. Mehta NM, Bechard LJ, Zurakowski D, et al. Adequate enteral protein intake is inversely associated to 60-d mortality in critically ill children: a multicenter, prospective cohort study. Am J Clin Nutr 2015;102:199–206.
58. Secker DJ, Jeejeebhoy KN. Subjective global nutritional assessment for children. Am J Clin Nutr 2007;85:1083–9.
59. Vermilyea S, Slicker J, El-Chammas K, et al. Subjective global nutritional assessment in critically ill children. J Parenter Enteral Nutr 2013;37(5):659–66.
60. Saggese G, Baroncelli GI. Bone status in children and adolescents with growth hormone deficiency: effect of growth hormone treatment. Int J Clin Pract Suppl 2002;126:18–21.
61. Van der Sluis IM, Boot AM, Hop WC, et al. Long-term effects of growth hormone therapy on bone mineral density, body composition, and serum lipid levels in growth hormone deficient children: a 6-year follow-up study. Horm Res 2002; 58:207–14.
62. Ali O, Shim M, Fowler E, et al. Growth hormone therapy improves bone mineral density in children with cerebral palsy: a preliminary pilot study. J Clin Endocrinol Metab 2007;92:932–7.
63. Ward K, Alsop C, Caulton J, et al. Low magnitude mechanical loading is osteogenic in children with disabling conditions. J Bone Miner Res 2004;19(3):360–9.
64. Ruck J, Chabot G, Rauch F. Vibration treatment in cerebral palsy: a randomized controlled pilot study. J Musculoskelet Neuronal Interact 2010;10(1):77–83.
65. Duquette SA, Guiliano AM, Starmer DJ. Whole body vibration and cerebral palsy: a systematic review. J Can Chiropr Assoc 2015;59(3):245–52.

Musculoskeletal Imaging in Cerebral Palsy

Katherine M. Schroeder, MD, John A. Heydemann, MD, Dorothy H. Beauvais, MD*

KEYWORDS

- Cerebral palsy • Radiographs • Hip surveillance • Scoliosis
- Knee flexion contracture • Flatfoot • Lower extremity deformities
- Limb length discrepancy

KEY POINTS

- Scoliosis, hip dysplasia, and other lower extremity deformities are commonly seen in patients with cerebral palsy. Plain radiographs are adequate for screening and diagnosis of these musculoskeletal issues.
- It is recommended that PA and lateral radiographs be obtained in a consistent fashion at least yearly but more often biannually for evaluation of scoliosis. The classic presentation of scoliosis associated with cerebral palsy is a long, C-shaped levokyphoscoliosis.
- Hip surveillance is important for screening for hip displacement in children with cerebral palsy and is done by measuring the hips migration percentage on an AP pelvis radiograph. Migration percentage greater than 30% warrants orthopedic evaluation.
- Rotational abnormalities, such as femoral anteversion, femoral retroversion, and tibial torsion, can contribute to gait dysfunction. Physical examination is commonly the first step in evaluation. Advanced imaging, such as MRI and CT scan, can provide additional information for preoperative planning.
- Leg length discrepancies and coronal plane deformities are best measured with standing teloroentgenograph (telegram).

INTRODUCTION

Scoliosis, hip dysplasia, and other lower extremity deformities are common musculoskeletal pathology found in patients with cerebral palsy. Imaging studies allow for an improved understanding of the pathology and can aid in planning treatment strategies. Most of these deformities in patients with cerebral palsy are visualized using plain radiographic techniques and occasionally require advanced imaging, such as computerized topography and MRI. The goal is to provide

Disclosure Statement: The authors have nothing to disclose.
Division of Pediatric Orthopaedic Surgery, Texas Children's Hospital, 6701 Fannin Street, Suite 660, Houston, TX 77030, USA
* Corresponding author.
E-mail address: dyharri1@texaschildrens.org

Phys Med Rehabil Clin N Am 31 (2020) 39–56
https://doi.org/10.1016/j.pmr.2019.09.001

insight into the various imaging techniques to better care for patients with cerebral palsy.

SPINE IMAGING

The overall incidence of scoliosis in patients with cerebral palsy is approximately 20%.[1] However, it is reported that patients with total body involvement can have an incidence of scoliosis up to 62% and bedridden children approaching 100%.[1–3] This was analyzed more thoroughly by Lee and colleagues.[4] They found that patients with Gross Motor Function Classification System (GMFCS) IV-V progression were noted to be 3.4° and 2.2° per year, respectively. Spinal deformities can present as scoliosis, kyphosis, lordosis, and pelvic obliquity.[1] The classic presentation is a long, C-shaped levokyphoscoliosis; however, other curve types do occur in more functional individuals.[5] Curve progression is noted to be gradual with rapid progression around the time of puberty, or when patients develop worsening function, or increased time spent in a wheelchair.[1] In addition, the larger the curve, the more likely it is to progress. This does not cease after skeletal maturity, because Thometz and Simon[6] noted that even after skeletal maturity curves less than 50° progressed. Assessment of the spine is initiated with the physical examination and subsequently confirmed with imaging studies.

There is no true consensus regarding the frequency and technique of imaging; however, it is recommended that radiographs be obtained in a consistent fashion at least yearly but more often biannually.[1,7] Plain posteroanterior and lateral complete spine 36-inch radiographs are obtained in a standing position (when possible) or sitting if the patient is unable to stand (**Figs. 1** and **2**).[7] Some centers use a standardized sitting frame with lateral support straps to ensure that there is minimal external support.[8] Furthermore, supine bending and traction films are obtained to assess flexibility (**Fig. 3**).[1,7] Should there be any suspicion of intraspinal pathology, Magnetic Resonance Imaging (MRI) is recommended. This may be observed as rapid progression at a young age, or change in neurologic status.[7] Scoliosis is measured on posteroanterior radiographs using the Cobb method.

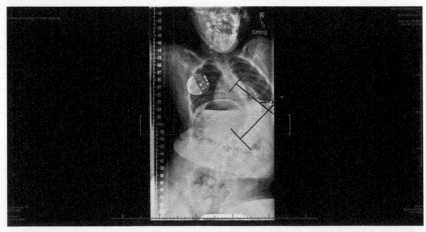

Fig. 1. Sitting posteroanterior plain radiograph demonstrating the Cobb measurement for evaluation of scoliosis.

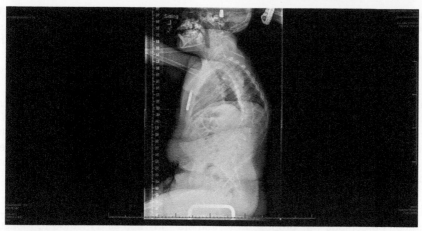

Fig. 2. Sitting lateral plain radiograph to evaluate for kyphosis or lordosis.

This consists of three steps by locating the superior end vertebra (or vertebra that is at the end of the curve), locating the inferior end vertebra, and drawing intersecting perpendicular lines. The angle of deviation of these perpendicular lines is the angle of the curve (see **Fig. 1**).[9] Scoliosis is considered to be a curve greater than 10°. In the sagittal plane, the cervical spine is lordotic, the thoracic spine is kyphotic (20°–50°), and the lumbar spine is lordotic (31°–79°). Kyphosis of the thoracic spine greater than 50° is considered abnormal.[9]

HIP IMAGING
Introduction and Incidence

Hip displacement and dislocation are commonly seen in children with cerebral palsy and results from spasticity and contracture of hip adductors, hip flexors, and medial hamstrings.[10] The incidence of hip displacement in children with cerebral palsy has

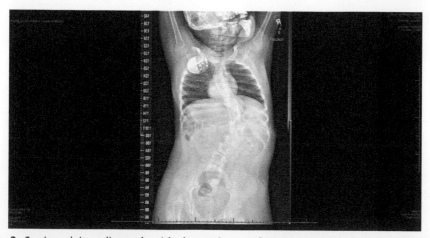

Fig. 3. Supine plain radiograph with the patient undergoing manual traction to demonstrate flexibility of the child's scoliosis.

been shown to have a linear relationship with level of gross motor function, with 0% for children with GMFCS level I to 90% for those with GMFCS level V.[10,11] Approximately 60% of children who are not walking by 5 years of age are likely to develop hip subluxation.[12]

Hip Surveillance

The success of surveillance programs to identify hip subluxation in children with cerebral palsy has been well established.[12–14] These programs rely on a combination of physical examination and radiographs, with the used of an anteroposterior (AP) pelvis radiograph.[13,15] The American Academy for Cerebral Palsy and Developmental Medicine has published a care pathway for hip surveillance (http://www.aacpdm.org/publications/care-pathways/hip-surveillance).[16]

Hip Radiographs

Migration percentage was proposed by Reimers[17] in 1980 as a method to measure the lateral displacement of the femoral head in children with cerebral palsy and has shown to have excellent intraobserver and interobserver reliability when performed correctly.[16] An AP pelvis radiograph is used to measure the migration percentage of hips. The proximal femurs should be posited in neutral abduction/adduction. Many children with cerebral palsy have increased lumbar lordosis and this should be corrected before imaging. This may be done by elevating the legs with a bump until the lower back is flush with the table and the lordosis is removed.

Migration percentage is measured as follows (**Fig. 4**):

1. Draw Hilgenreiner line (H) horizontally between the superior aspects of the triradiate cartilages. After skeletal maturity, the inferior points of the acetabular teardrops may be used.
2. Draw Perkin line (P), perpendicular to the Hilgenreiner line, at the lateral edge of each acetabulum.
3. Draw lines parallel to Perkin line, along the medial and lateral extent of each femoral head.

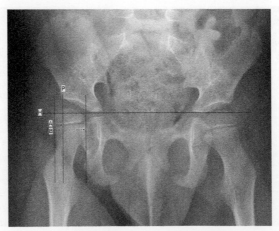

Fig. 4. Hip migration percentage. Migration percentage is calculated as a percentage of A/B. H, Hilgenreiner line; P, Perkin line.

4. Measure the width of the femoral head (B).
5. Measure the distance between Perkin line and the lateral aspect of the femoral head (A).
6. Calculate migration percentage: A/B × 100%.

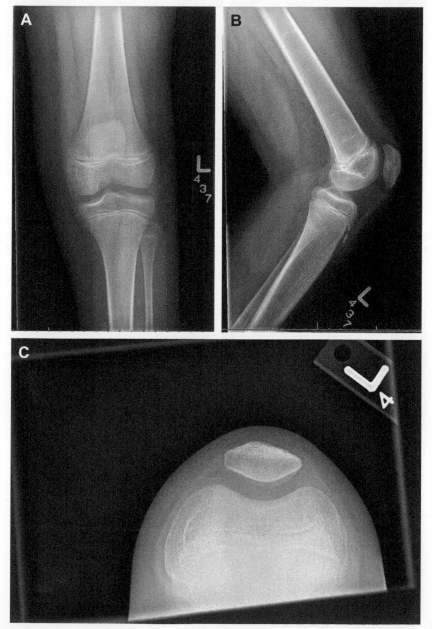

Fig. 5. A 10-year-old girl with right hemiplegic cerebral palsy; unaffected left side shown to demonstrate normal AP (*A*), 30° lateral (*B*), and sunrise view (*C*).

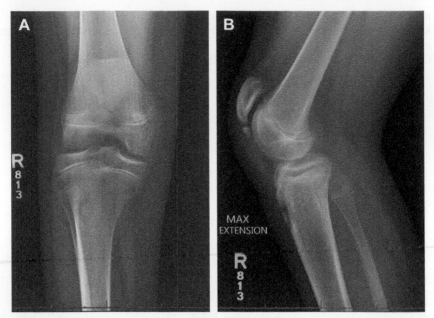

Fig. 6. A 12-year-old boy with diplegic cerebral palsy, GMFCS II; AP and maximum extension lateral shown. (*A*) AP view of the knee. (*B*) Maximum extension lateral of the knee. Note patella alta, patellar pole fracture/fragmentation and flexion contracture on maximum extension lateral (*B*).

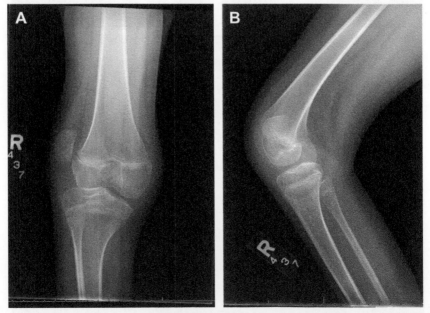

Fig. 7. An 11-year-old girl, quadriplegic, GMFCS IV with painful lateral subluxation of her patella. (*A*) AP Image of the knee with laterally displaced patella. (*B*) 30 degree lateral of the knee with dislocated patella.

In general, a referral to a pediatric orthopedic surgeon is recommended if the migration percentage is greater than 30% or the patient has less than 30° of hip abduction on physical examination.[17]

KNEE IMAGING

The knee is a source of pain and gait dysfunction in patients with cerebral palsy. Common problems include anterior knee pain, patella subluxation/dislocations, inferior patellar pole fractures, patella alta, and knee flexion contractures.[5,8,18,19] Radiographic imaging is necessary to assess and diagnosis knee deformities and provide important information for surgical planning.

Standard radiographic evaluation of the knee includes three views: an AP, a 30° lateral, and a sunrise view (**Fig. 5**). The sunrise view is particularly necessary when there are concerns of patellar subluxation/dislocation or patellar maltracking. The

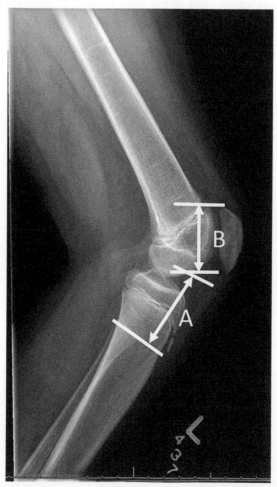

Fig. 8. Insall-Salvati ratio: A/B: ratio between the lengths of the patellar tendon (A), from its origin at the inferior pole of the patella to its insertion at the tibial tubercle, and the length of the patella (B) from the superior pole to the inferior pole.

30° lateral view is used to assess inferior patellar pole fractures and patella alta (**Figs. 6** and **7**). Several methods exists for assessing patellar height and defining patella alta.

The Insall-Salvati Index, the Koshino Index, and the Caton-Deschamps are the most frequently used in cerebral palsy. The Insall-Salvati index, although developed for adults, has been shown to have high validity with MRI patellar tendon lengths in healthy children.[20,21] Furthermore, in boys greater than 12 and girls greater than 10 the Insall-Salvati method approximates that of a skeletally mature knee (**Fig. 8**).[18,20] The Koshino index has been used previously in patients with cerebral palsy to assess outcomes following patellar tendon shortening surgery[22–24] and has been shown to be stable throughout a range of knee flexion from 30° to 90° with normal being 0.9 to 1.3 (**Fig. 9**).[18,25] The Caton-Deschamps index[26] has been proposed as a simpler method to the Insall-Salvati index and the Koshino index for the evaluation of children and adolescents (**Fig. 10**).[27]

For patients with crouch gait or concern for knee flexion contractures, a maximum extension lateral view of the knee is used to determine the degree of

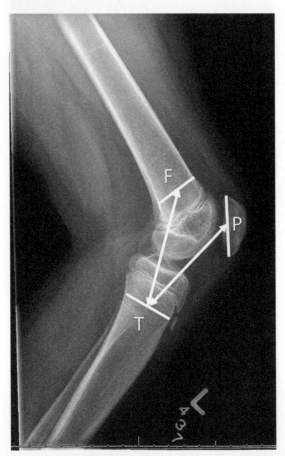

Fig. 9. Koshino index: PT/FT is measured as the ratio between the patella-tibia (PT) and femur-tibia (FT) distance using the mid-epiphyseal points. Note there are different anatomic landmarks depending on the age of the patient.

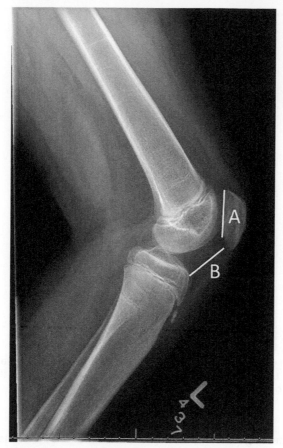

Fig. 10. Caton-Deschamps index (B/A): ratio between the joint surface of the patella to the anterosuperior angle of the tibia (B) to the length of the patellar articular surface (A).

contracture. This view is obtained by placing a bolster beneath the ankle and asking the patient to extend at the knee; if patients are not able to actively extend, an assistant can hold the leg in maximum extension. There is no standardized technique for measuring knee flexion contractures. Common techniques include measuring the angle between the mid-diaphyseal points of the femoral shaft and mid-diaphyseal points of the tibial shaft; or measuring the angle between the anterior femoral shaft cortex and the posterior tibial shaft cortex (**Fig 11**).

FOOT AND ANKLE IMAGING

Foot and ankle disorders are common in patients in cerebral palsy and can cause pain and difficulty with orthotic wear and hinder efficient gait. Common disorders include ankle valgus, equinus, equinovarus, equinovalgus, and planovalgus deformities.[28] Radiographic evaluation is helpful in evaluating complaints of pain, confirming deformity, and preparing for surgical correction. Standard foot series

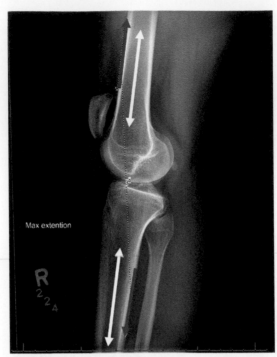

Fig. 11. Maximum extension lateral. Angle between with anterior femoral cortex and posterior tibial cortex (*red arrow*) or the angle between the mid-diaphysis of the femur and the mid-diaphysis of the tibia (*white arrow*).

include weight-bearing (when possible) AP, lateral, and oblique views of the foot. Typically, the AP and lateral are sufficient for evaluation. If there is concern for ankle valgus, a weight-bearing AP and mortise view of the ankle can assess the distal tibia alignment (**Fig. 12**).

Normative values for pediatric foot alignment have been defined.[29,30] On a weight-bearing AP film, forefoot and hindfoot alignment are assessed through the talo–first metatarsal angle and the talocalcaneal angle, respectively (**Figs. 13–15**). The reported normal range for the AP talus–first metatarsal angle is $6° \pm 7°$ according to Vanderwilde and colleagues[30] and $10° \pm 7°$ according to Davids.[29] The greater the AP talo–first metatarsal angle the more abducted the foot. The reported normal range for the AP talocalcaneal angle is from $10°$ to $56°$. The measurement of the AP talocalcaneal has been noted to be unreliable and difficult to measure because of poor visualization hindfoot on standard AP films. Lastly, on the AP view the coverage of the talar head by the navicular is assessed (see **Fig. 13**C). Lateral subluxation of the navicular on the head of the talus is seen in valgus foot deformities, whereas, medial subluxation is noted in varus deformities. Davids[29] developed the talonavicular coverage angle to further quantify the degree of subluxation with normal values $20° \pm 9.8°$. Values greater than this indicate midfoot abduction.

On the lateral radiograph, angles of importance include the talocalcaneal angle, the talus–first metatarsal angle, and the tibiocalcaneal angle (or calcaneal pitch angle). The lateral talocalcaneal angle is used to assess hindfoot alignment.

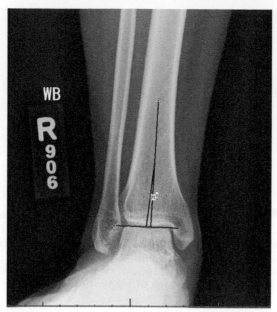

Fig. 12. An 18-year-old spastic diplegic GMFCS II. Normal distal tibial alignment. Shown is the measurement for the lateral distal tibia angle measured along the anatomic axis. Normal is 89° (86–92) (Mosca).

Normal reported values are 49±6.9[29] and 39±7.[30] The greater the angle, indicates a more abducted and valgus hindfoot, whereas smaller angles indicate a more varus and adducted hindfoot (**Figs. 16–18**). The lateral talus–first metatarsal angle is a measurement of midfoot deformity with normal values of 13 ± 7.5 and 8 ± 6. When the first metatarsal is dorsiflexed relative to the talus the value is

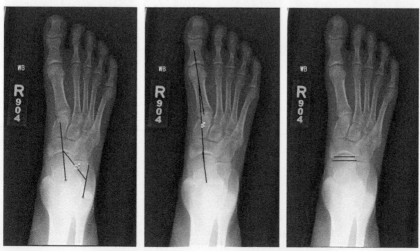

Fig. 13. Normal AP image of a foot demonstrating the AP talocalcaneal angle (A), the AP talo–first metatarsal angle (B), and the talonavicular coverage angle (C).

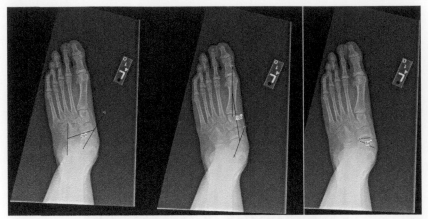

Fig. 14. AP foot in a 13-year-old GMFCS III diplegic boy with flat foot deformity of the left foot. Note the medial deviation of the talar head and increased talocalcaneal angle (*Left*). The increased talo–first metatarsal angle indicated forefoot abduction (*Middle*) and the increased talonavicular coverage angle because of medial deviation of the talus and abduction of the forefoot leading to uncoverage of the talar head (*Right*).

positive. The larger the angle the more planus the midfoot. Conversely, when the first metatarsal is plantarflex relative to the talus the value is negative and indicates a cavus midfoot (see **Fig. 18**). Equinus or plantarflexion deformity is assessed through the tibiocalcaneal angle or the calcaneal pitch. Reported normal values of the tibiocalcaneal angle are 69° ± 8.4°[29] and 39° ± 7.[30] For the calcaneal pitch, the range is 17° ± 6°[29] and 22°[30] (11°–38°). The angles are increased in equinus and plantarflexion deformities and decreased in calcaneus and dorsiflexion deformities.

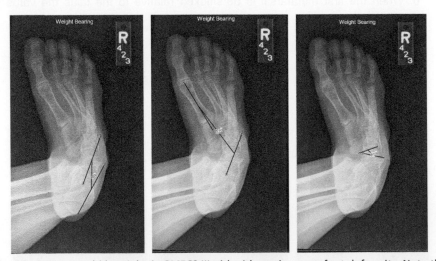

Fig. 15. A 12-year-old hemiplegic GMFCS III girl with equinovarus foot deformity. Note the decreased AP talocalcaneal angle because of hindfoot varus (*Left*). There is lateral deviation of the talar head resulting in a negative talo–first metatarsal angle (*Middle*). There is undercoverage of the talar head (*Right*).

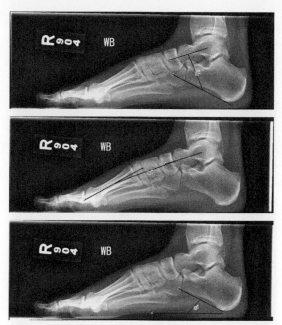

Fig. 16. Normal lateral of the foot demonstrating the lateral talocalcaneal angle (*top*), the lateral talo-first metatarsal angle (*middle*), and the calcaneal pitch (*bottom*).

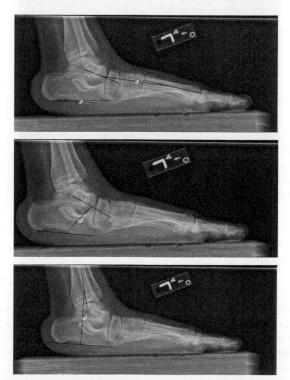

Fig. 17. Lateral foot in a 13-year-old GMFCS III diplegic boy with flat foot deformity of the left foot. There is apex plantar deviation of the lateral talo-first metatarsal angle and decreased calcaneal pitch (*top*). The lateral talocalcaneal angle is increased (*middle*). The lateral tibiocalcaneal angle is increased (*bottom*).

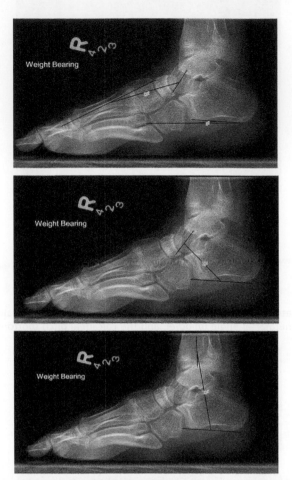

Fig. 18. Lateral weight bearing radiograph of a 12 year old hemiplegic girl with equinovarus foot deformity. The lateral talo-first metatarsal angle and calcaneal pitch are abnormal (*top*). The lateral talo-calcaneal angle is decreased indicating hindfoot varus (*middle*). The tibiocalcaneal angle is increased indicating equinus (*bottom*).

IMAGING FOR ROTATIONAL ABNORMALITIES, LEG LENGTH DISCREPANCY, AND CORONAL DEFORMITIES
Rotational Abnormalities

Rotational abnormalities are common in children with cerebral palsy and can contribute to gait difficulty in ambulatory patients.[31,32] Although femoral anteversion (or internal hip rotation) is the most common rotational abnormality, femoral anteversion and femoral retroversion along with internal and external tibial torsion have been described in children with cerebral palsy.[31] Although physical examination and observation of the patient's gait pattern should be the first evaluation of such rotational abnormalities, advanced imaging can provide additional information and is used for preoperative planning. Both MRI and computed tomography may be used for cross-sectional imaging. Images are obtained at the femoral neck, femoral condyles, tibial plateau, and ankle.[33] Alternatively, EOS 2D/3D low-dose digital imaging device (EOS Imaging SA, Paris, France) can provide images that may be manipulated to all for two-dimensional and three-dimensional evaluation of lower extremity rotation.[34] Femoral version is determined by measuring the angle between two lines: one parallel to the femoral neck and the other parallel to the posterior femoral condyles. Tibial torsion is measured similarly, with one line parallel the tibial plateau and the other parallel the posterior aspects of the medial and lateral malleoli.[35]

Leg Length Discrepancy and Coronal Deformities

Leg length inequality is most often seen in children with hemiplegic cerebral palsy and can contribute to gait abnormalities in this population.[36] Radiographically, the most basic way to measure a leg length inequality is via orthoroentgenography (also called a scanogram), where images at the hip, knee, and ankle are taken onto a single large cassette, along with an opaque ruler. Conversely, teloroentgenography (also called a teleogram) is taken using a single exposure on a long film with the tube detector 6 feet away from the patient.[35] If there is a significant leg length inequality, an appropriately sized block should be placed the short foot, to clinically level the pelvis before taking the teleogram. Furthermore, EOS 2D/3D low-dose imaging is used to determine leg length (**Fig. 19**).[34]

Although less common than rotational abnormalities and leg length inequality, coronal deformities of the lower extremities can also be seen in children with cerebral

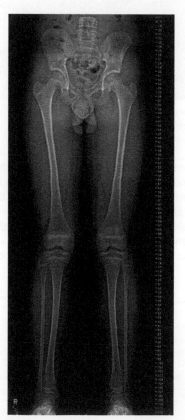

Fig. 19. An example of a teleogram performed on an EOS 2D/3D low-dose imaging device. This 14-year-old boy has no significant leg length discrepancy.

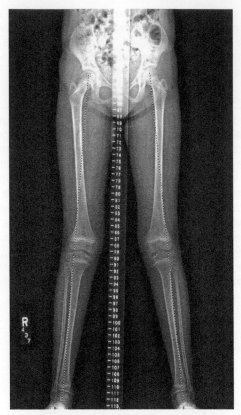

Fig. 20. Teleogram of a 6-year-old boy showing the mechanical axis of both knees falling in the lateral third of the knee joints, indicating genu valgum.

palsy. The previously mentioned scanogram is the ideal modality to assess coronal deformity, particularly genu varum and genu valgum. A line indicating the mechanical axis of the leg is drawn from the center of the femoral head to the center of the ankle.[37] When the leg is in neutral alignment, the mechanical axis should fall though the center third of the knee. Valgus alignment is noted when this line falls in the lateral third of the knee joint or lateral to the knee (**Fig. 20**). Conversely, varus alignment is noted when the mechanical axis falls through the medial third of the knee joint or medial to the knee.

REFERENCES

1. McCarthy JJ, D'Andrea LP, Betz RR, et al. Scoliosis in the child with cerebral palsy. J Am Acad Orthop Surg 2006;14(6):367–75.

2. Hodgkinson I, Bérard C, Chotel F, et al. Pelvic obliquity and scoliosis in non-ambulatory patients with cerebral palsy: a descriptive study of 234 patients over 15 years of age. Rev Chir Orthop Reparatrice Appar Mot 2002;88(4): 337–41 [in French].

3. Saito N, Ebara S, Ohotsuka K, et al. Natural history of scoliosis in spastic cerebral palsy. Lancet 1998;351(9117):1687–92.

4. Lee SY, Chung CY, Lee KM, et al. Annual changes in radiographic indices of the spine in cerebral palsy patients. Eur Spine J 2016;25(3):679–86.

5. Chan G, Miller F. Assessment and treatment of children with cerebral palsy. Orthop Clin North Am 2014;45(3):313–25.

6. Thometz JG, Simon SR. Progression of scoliosis after skeletal maturity in institutionalized adults who have cerebral palsy. J Bone Joint Surg Am 1988;70(9): 1290–6.

7. Akbarnia BA, Yazici M, Thompson GH. The growing spine: management of spinal disorders in young children. 2nd edition. Berlin: Springer; 2016.

8. Miller F. Cerebral palsy. New York: Springer; 2005. Publisher description. Available at: http://www.loc.gov/catdir/enhancements/fy0662/2003065734-d.html http://www.loc.gov/catdir/enhancements/fy0818/2003065734-t.html.

9. Canale ST, Beaty JH, Campbell WCOo. Campbell's operative orthopaedics. Philadelphia (PA): Elsevier/Mosby; 2013.

10. Soo B, Howard JJ, Boyd RN, et al. Hip displacement in cerebral palsy. J Bone Joint Surg Am 2006;88(1):121–9.

11. Pruszczynski B, Sees J, Miller F. Risk factors for hip displacement in children with cerebral palsy: systematic review. J Pediatr Orthop 2016;36(8):829–33.

12. Gordon GS, Simkiss DE. A systematic review of the evidence for hip surveillance in children with cerebral palsy. J Bone Joint Surg Br 2006;88(11):1492–6.

13. Hägglund G, Alriksson-Schmidt A, Lauge-Pedersen H, et al. Prevention of dislocation of the hip in children with cerebral palsy: 20-year results of a population-based prevention programme. Bone Joint J 2014;96-B(11):1546–52.

14. Wynter M, Gibson N, Willoughby KL, et al. Australian hip surveillance guidelines for children with cerebral palsy: 5-year review. Dev Med Child Neurol 2015;57(9): 808–20.

15. Hägglund G, Lauge-Pedersen H, Persson M. Radiographic threshold values for hip screening in cerebral palsy. J Child Orthop 2007;1(1):43–7.

16. Cliffe L, Sharkey D, Charlesworth G, et al. Correct positioning for hip radiographs allows reliable measurement of hip displacement in cerebral palsy. Dev Med Child Neurol 2011;53(6):549–52.

17. Mayson T, Miller S, Cairns R, et al. Hip surveillance: bottom line 'evidence-informed' recommendations for the hip surveillance in individuals with cerebral palsy. 2017. Available at: http://www.aacpdm.org/publications/care-pathways/hip-surveillance. Accessed March 9, 2019.

18. Gage JR. The identification and treatment of gait problems in cerebral palsy. 2nd edition. London: Mac Keith Press : Distributed by Wiley-Blackwell; 2009.

19. Senaran H, Holden C, Dabney KW, et al. Anterior knee pain in children with cerebral palsy. J Pediatr Orthop 2007;27(1):12–6.

20. Insall J, Salvati E. Patella position in the normal knee joint. Radiology 1971;101(1): 101–4.

21. Park MS, Chung CY, Lee KM, et al. Which is the best method to determine the patellar height in children and adolescents? Clin Orthop Relat Res 2010;468(5): 1344–51.

22. Hösl M, Böhm H, Seltmann M, et al. Relationship between radiographic patella-alta pathology and walking dysfunction in children with bilateral spastic cerebral palsy. Gait Posture 2018;60:28–34.

23. Sossai R, Vavken P, Brunner R, et al. Patellar tendon shortening for flexed knee gait in spastic diplegia. Gait Posture 2015;41(2):658–65.

24. Stout JL, Gage JR, Schwartz MH, et al. Distal femoral extension osteotomy and patellar tendon advancement to treat persistent crouch gait in cerebral palsy. J Bone Joint Surg Am 2008;90(11):2470–84.

25. Novacheck TF, Stout JL, Gage JR, et al. Distal femoral extension osteotomy and patellar tendon advancement to treat persistent crouch gait in cerebral palsy. Surgical technique. J Bone Joint Surg Am 2009;91(Suppl 2):271–86.

26. Caton J, Deschamps G, Chambat P, et al. Les rotules basses: a propos de 128 observations. Rev Chir Orthop Reparatrice Appar Mot 1982;68:317–25.

27. Thévenin-Lemoine C, Ferrand M, Courvoisier A, et al. Is the Caton-Deschamps index a valuable ratio to investigate patellar height in children? J Bone Joint Surg Am 2011;93(8):e35.

28. Davids JR. The foot and ankle in cerebral palsy. Orthop Clin North Am 2010;41: 579–93.

29. Davids JR. Biomechanically based clinical decision making in pediatric foot and ankle surgery. In: Sabharwal S, editor. Pediatric lower limb deformities: principles and techniques of management. 1st edition. Cham (Switzerland): Springer; 2016. p. 153–63.

30. Vanderwilde R, Staheli LT, Chew DE, et al. Measurements on radiographs of the foot in normal infants and children. J Bone Joint Surg Am 1988;70(3):407–15.

31. Aktas S, Aiona MD, Orendurff M. Evaluation of rotational gait abnormality in the patients cerebral palsy. J Pediatr Orthop 2000;20(2):217–20.

32. van der Linden ML, Hazlewood ME, Hillman SJ, et al. Passive and dynamic rotation of the lower limbs in children with diplegic cerebral palsy. Dev Med Child Neurol 2006;48(3):176–80.

33. Koenig JK, Pring ME, Dwek JR. MR evaluation of femoral neck version and tibial torsion. Pediatr Radiol 2012;42(1):113–5.

34. Wybier M, Bossard P. Musculoskeletal imaging in progress: the EOS imaging system. Joint Bone Spine 2013;80(3):238–43.

35. Stein-Wexler R, Wootton-Gorges SL, Ozonoff MB. Pediatric orthopedic imaging. Heidelberg (Germany): Springer; 2015.

36. Allen PE, Jenkinson A, Stephens MM, et al. Abnormalities in the uninvolved lower limb in children with spastic hemiplegia: the effect of actual and functional leg-length discrepancy. J Pediatr Orthop 2000;20(1):88–92.

37. Vaishya R, Vijay V, Birla VP, et al. Inter-observer variability and its correlation to experience in measurement of lower limb mechanical axis on long leg radiographs. J Clin Orthop Trauma 2016;7(4):260–4.

Medical Updates in Management of Hypertonia

Rochelle Dy, MD[a],*, Desiree Roge, MD[b]

KEYWORDS

- Hypertonia • Spasticity • Dystonia • Chemodenervation • Botulinum toxin • Phenol
- Goal setting

KEY POINTS

- There is not enough evidence for the efficacy of oral agents in the treatment of hypertonia in children.
- Chemodenervation is an adjunct in the treatment of hypertonia.
- Management of hypertonia should be multimodal, with shared family goals set to improve function, quality of life, activity, and participation.

Cerebral palsy (CP) has been defined as a disorder of movement and motor control that results from a nonprogressive injury to the fetal or infant brain. CP is the most common motor disability in childhood. Hypertonic CP is the most common form of CP, accounting for more than 80% of cases.

A review of the different terms defines hypertonia as abnormally increased resistance to externally imposed movement about a joint. It may be caused by spasticity, dystonia, rigidity, or a combination of features. Spasticity is hypertonia in which resistance to externally imposed movement increases with increasing speed of stretch and varies with the direction of joint movement. Dystonia is a movement disorder in which involuntary sustained or intermittent muscle contractions cause twisting and repetitive movements, abnormal postures, or both. Rigidity is a bidirectional resistance throughout the range of motion that may involve simultaneous cocontraction of agonists and antagonists. It is independent of velocity.[1]

Identifying the subtypes of hypertonia is becoming increasingly important. Treatment strategies, including tone-modulating surgical interventions, and medication type and dosing, may differ depending on the type of hypertonia present. The Hypertonia Assessment Tool (HAT) is a 7-item clinical assessment tool used to differentiate the various types of pediatric hypertonia. It was validated and published in 2010. This tool has shown good reliability and validity for identifying spasticity and the absence of rigidity, and moderate findings for identifying dystonia.[2] Treatment of hypertonia is

[a] PM&R, Texas Children's Hospital, 6701 Fannin Street, Suite D1280, Houston, TX 77030, USA;
[b] Seattle Children's Hospital, 4800 Sand Point Way NE, Seattle, WA 98105, USA
* Corresponding author.
E-mail address: rtdy@texaschildrens.org

Phys Med Rehabil Clin N Am 31 (2020) 57–68
https://doi.org/10.1016/j.pmr.2019.09.010
1047-9651/20/© 2019 Elsevier Inc. All rights reserved.

more successful when delivered by an interdisciplinary team that understands the unique challenges that arise in managing and treating children with CP. Unlike adults, children with hypertonia develop growth-related musculoskeletal deformities. These deformities include joint contraction and lever arm deformities, which in the long term may affect function and participation in a negative way. Health care providers who care for children with CP understand that not all hypertonia needs to be treated. There are benefits related to having underlying hypertonia in patients with a neurologic motor impairment that can translate to function. Management of hypertonia has evolved through the years. Emphasis now is to promote changes in activity and participation, in addition to caregiver goals of care and comfort.

This article reviews oral pharmacologic agents and chemodenervation.

ORAL PHARMACOLOGY
Pharmacologic Management for Spasticity

Generalized hypertonia is often treated with oral medications. Various oral agents have been reported to decrease spasticity; none have been proved to improve function. The most common medications used to treat spasticity include enteral baclofen, diazepam, clonazepam, clonidine, tizanidine, and dantrolene. With the exception of dantrolene, these medications work at the central nervous system (CNS). The side effects profile includes sedation and drowsiness, which may limit titration to therapeutic doses. Most oral medications can be used in combination.

Diazepam and clonazepam are benzodiazepines and belong to the anticonvulsants. Benzodiazepines facilitate CNS inhibition via potentiation of gamma-aminobutyric acid (GABA) at the spinal and supraspinal levels, leading to a reduction in spasticity, hyperreflexia, and muscle spasms. Side effects include sedation, difficulty with consolidation and formation of memory, urinary retention, liver toxicity, and dependency.[3] There is limited number of studies available on the efficacy of benzodiazepines in the treatment of hypertonia in children. In 2010, the American Academy of Neurology published a practice parameter on the pharmacologic treatment of spasticity in children and adolescents with CP. Diazepam was recommended for the short-term treatment of spasticity in children with CP. The benefits of diazepam were dose dependent and included tone reduction, increased passive range of motion, and increase in spontaneous movements. There was no evidence to support improvement in function.[3]

Baclofen works presynaptically and postsynaptically as a GABA B agonist. It crosses the blood-brain barrier and binds to GABA B receptors in the spinal cord. It inhibits the release of excitatory neurotransmitters.[4] The side effects of baclofen include sedation, confusion, dizziness, ataxia, weakness, nausea, and hypotension.[5] Oral baclofen is generally used as first-line treatment of spasticity and dystonia because it is less sedating than other medications, such as the benzodiazepine group. Pharmacokinetic studies in children with CP suggest that oral baclofen dosage can be based on body weight (BW) (2 mg/kg/d) in children with CP older than 2 years.[6]

The most recent systematic review was conducted in 2016 and it assessed the effectiveness of oral baclofen in the treatment of spasticity in children and adolescents with CP. It concluded that there are insufficient data to support or refute the use of oral baclofen for reducing spasticity or improving motor function in children and adolescents with CP.[7,8]

In 2018, McLaughlin and colleagues[9] studied the pharmacogenomic variability of oral baclofen and how it can contribute to differences in pharmacokinetics and clinical responses.

Although it was a small sample, there was evidence to suggest that specific allelic variants had better clinical response showing decreased spasticity. This finding means that there is a genetic variation that affects drug clearance, and therefore some children with CP may respond to this drug better than others.[9]

Tizanidine is a centrally acting alpha-2 noradrenergic agonist.[4] Alpha-2 adrenergic agonists also have an antinociceptive effect through the release of substance P in the spinal cord.[6] They are often used in conjunction with other oral agents, such as baclofen, for additive effects.[4] Side effects include hypotension, sedation, asthenia, dry mouth, dizziness, hallucination, and hepatotoxicity. It is also known to prolong QT interval.

Dantrolene works at the muscle level by inhibiting the release of calcium by the sarcoplasmic reticulum. In addition to reducing tone, it can lead to weakness and sedation despite its peripheral mechanism of action.[5] Other side effects include hepatotoxicity, nausea, vomiting, and diarrhea.

PHARMACOLOGIC MANAGEMENT OF DYSTONIA

There is limited information regarding prescription practices in childhood dystonia. Similar to spasticity management, the use of medications is limited by side effects. A systematic review published in 2017 on management of dystonia in children with CP concluded that there was insufficient evidence to support the use of any oral medication for the treatment of dystonia.[10]

The most common medications used for the treatment of dystonia include oral baclofen, levodopa, trihexyphenidyl, and the benzodiazepines diazepam and clonazepam.

Levodopa is a dopamine precursor that crosses the blood-brain barrier to produce central dopaminergic effects.[10] It is the first line of treatment for dopa-responsive dystonia. This property has led to its use in secondary dystonia such as that seen in children with CP.

There is no evidence that individuals with dystonic CP have a deficiency in dopaminergic transmission within the basal ganglia.[10] Pozin and colleagues[11] published a small randomized controlled trial of levodopa in children with dystonic CP who showed no significant improvement in function. The side effects of levodopa include gastrointestinal upset, nausea, hallucinations, dyskinesia, and drowsiness.

Trihexyphenidyl is a centrally acting anticholinergic agent. It has been postulated that it works by rebalancing the cholinergic to dopaminergic interneural drive in the basal ganglia.[10] Over the last 15 years there have been a few studies of the effectiveness of trihexyphenidyl in reducing dystonia and improving upper limb function in individuals with CP, while other studies have shown the opposite. A recent Cochrane Review, published in 2018, found that there is insufficient evidence to support trihexyphenidyl as being effective in reducing dystonia or improving function among individuals with CP.[12] The systematic review by Fehlings and colleagues[10] in 2018 concluded that trihexyphenidyl is possibly ineffective in reducing dystonia or improving function. Side effects of trihexyphenidyl include constipation, urinary retention, dry mouth, blurred vision, and behavior changes, therefore gradual dose escalation is recommended.

Gabapentin is an anticonvulsant. In the last few years it has been used primarily to improve pain and comfort in children. A recent retrospective observational study by Liow[13], published in 2016, investigated 69 children with severe dystonia of different causes, including 25 children with CP, and reported a significant decrease in the severity of dystonia and pain, and increased seating tolerance and quality and quantity of sleep.[13,14] It is typically well tolerated, with the most common side effect being sedation. A summary of commonly used oral medications for spasticity and dystonia with their respective dosing schedule is listed in **Table 1**.

MEDICAL MARIJUANA

Marijuana contains cannabinoids, which are pharmacologically active compounds. 9-Tetrahydrocannabinol (THC) and cannabidiol (CBD) are two of the compounds that have been isolated.

CB-1 and CB-2 are cannabinoid receptors that can be found in the brain and spinal cord. CB-1 receptors are concentrated in the hippocampus, basal ganglia, cerebellum, dorsal root ganglia in the spinal cord, and presynaptic sympathetic nerve endings in peripheral nerves, and CB-2 receptors can be found in the periaqueductal gray.[15] THC is responsible for symptoms of psychosis and well-being.

In the past few years the use of cannabinoids for the treatment of spasticity and dystonia has become more prevalent. However, there is insufficient evidence to justify its use in the management of children with spasticity or dystonia related to CP.[15,16] There is some evidence emerging in the management of spasticity associated with multiple sclerosis[15] and epilepsy.[16]

CHEMODENERVATION FOR SPASTICITY MANAGEMENT

Over the past 2 decades, chemodenervation with botulinum toxin (BoNT) has become an integral component of the clinician's toolbox in the management of focal or segmental spasticity and dystonia in children with CP. Its efficacy has been recognized in reducing spasticity and thereby preventing secondary musculoskeletal deformities and joint contractures and possibly delaying the need for surgery, decreasing hypertonia-related pain, providing better tolerance of splinting, improving hygiene, decreasing caregiver burden, facilitating function, and supporting motor development.[17,18] However, spasticity is only 1 of the components in the upper motor neuron syndrome. Muscle weakness, impaired motor planning and control, coordination, and muscle strength regulation contribute to the overall impairment of motor function and must be equally considered when formulating the treatment goal.[19,20]

Topographic descriptions of affected limbs and classifications of motor function in CP provide a good familiarization with the typical movement patterns and muscle groups commonly affected. However, the degree and severity of involvement, distribution of weakness, and motor abilities vary from one person to another, thus the need for specialized and individualized treatment cannot be overemphasized.

It is common for oral/systemic pharmacologic intervention to be needed in conjunction with BoNT treatment, particularly in children and adolescents with mixed-type hypertonia. BoNT is not to be used in isolation but as an adjunct to achieving goals through a multimodal approach in conjunction with other treatment modalities, such as therapeutic exercise with physical and occupational therapy, splinting/bracing, and serial casting.[20–22]

BOTULINUM TOXINS

There are currently 7 serotypes of BoNT, A to G, but only serotypes A and B are clinically used for therapeutic treatment. These serotypes are purified neurotoxins from fermentation of the *Clostridium botulinum* bacteria. Once injected intramuscularly, the toxin is taken up at the peripheral cholinergic nerve endings to cleave SNARE (SNAP-25 in BoNT-A; synaptobrevin in BoNT-B) proteins, preventing acetylcholine

Table 1
Oral medications for management of spasticity/dystonia

Use	Generic Name	Dosage	Mechanism of Action	Side Effects
Spasticity/ dystonia	Baclofen	Start 2.5 mg TID, maximum dose 80 mg/d divided TID in children >8 y/o	GABA B agonist	Sedation (but less than benzodiazepines), constipation
Spasticity/ dystonia	Clonazepam	0.01–0.3 mg/kg/d divided BID or TID	GABA A agonist	Sedation, drooling, constipation
Spasticity	Clonidine	Start at 0.05 mg/d and increase by 0.05 mg every week to a maximum of 0.3 mg/d divided TID	Central-acting alpha-2 adrenergic agonists	Sedation, hypotension, bradycardia
Spasticity/ dystonia	Dantrolene	0.5 mg/kg divided BID, increase every week to a maximum of 12 mg/kg/d divided QID	Interferes with release of calcium from sarcoplasmic reticulum in skeletal muscles	Weakness, sedation (but less than others), hepatotoxicity
Spasticity/ dystonia	Diazepam	0.05–0.1 mg/kg/d divided BID to QID	GABA A agonist	Sedation, constipation, urinary retention
Spasticity	Gabapentin	Start 10–15 mg/kg/d divided TID, titrate maximum of 60 mg/kg/d divided TID	Unknown	Sedation, emotional lability
Dystonia	Carbidopa/le vodopa	25/100: start 0.25–0.5 tablet BID, maximum 800 mg/d divided BID or TID	Dopamine precursor, indirect receptor agonist	Rarely effective in CP, more effective in genetic dystonia GI upset; may add extra carbidopa (Lodosyn) to alleviate side effects, sedation
Spasticity/ cramps	Tizanidine	Start 1–2 mg QHS with maintenance 0.3–0.5 mg/kg/d divided TID or QID	Central-acting alpha-2 adrenergic agonists	Sedation, hypotension, hepatotoxicity
Dystonia	Trihexyphenidyl	Start 2–2.5 mg/d, increase by 2–2.5 mg every other week to maximum dose of 60 mg/d divided BID or TID	Anticholinergic	Sedation, constipation, urinary retention, dry mouth, dyskinesias, motor tics

Abbreviations: BID, twice a day; GI, gastrointestinal; QHS, at bedtime; QID, 4 times a day; TID, 3 times a day.

vesicle docking and release into the neuromuscular junction, which results in muscle contraction inhibition. The effect of reduced muscle activation is temporary because transmission reoccurs gradually and new nerve endings are formed. The effect develops within 3 days after injection and may reach its peak effect from 10 to 30 days, lasting for 3 to 6 months.[23]

DOSING AND ADMINISTRATION

Table 2 lists the most commonly available BoNT preparations. Although licensing varies between different countries, the use of BoNT for spasticity treatment in children has generally been accepted as an off-label medication. Clinical trials on dosing in children are sparse or are generally of small sample size, and treatment guidelines remain unclear. Systematic reviews, consensus statements, and best-practice guidelines have been helpful references for treatment protocols, although there is still a need for vigilant observation toward further understanding of its effects among children with CP and other neurologic conditions with hypertonia.

OnabotulinumtoxinA (ONA) for spasticity in children with CP was first introduced by Koman [27] in 1993 using 5 U/kg BW. Over the years, several studies have proposed increasing doses of up to 20 to 25 U/kg BW. Concerns were raised with the report of the deaths of 4 children after receiving BoNT-A injection, which resulted in the US Food and Drug Administration (FDA) release of a black box warning in 2008 regarding potential for systemic spread leading to pulmonary distress and death. The 2010 international consensus statement recommends a lower range of dosing of 12 to 16 U/kg BW, particularly for patients of Gross Motor Function Classification System (GMFCS) level V, and any patient with dysphagia or breathing problems.[22,28]

Strobl and colleagues[20] recommend incobotulinumtoxinA (INCO) doses to start at less than or equal to 12 U/kg BW for the first injection, with subsequent injections of up to 15 U/kg BW, based on INCO's comparable efficacy, potency, and adverse event profile with ONA when using a clinical conversion ratio of 1:1.[26,29] AbobotulinumtoxinA (ABO) was approved by the FDA in 2016 for pediatric lower limb spasticity, for patients

Table 2 Botulinum toxins commonly used in cerebral palsy, dosage forms, and recommended dosing		
Botulinum Toxin Generic/Brand Names	**Dosage Form and Strength in the United States**	**Recommended Dosing**
AbobotulinumtoxinA (Dysport)	300-U vial 500-U vial	10–15 U/kg per limb maximum dose: 30 U/kg for bilateral injections or a total of 1000 U[24,25]
IncobotulinumtoxinA (Xeomin)	50-U vial 100-U vial 200-U vial	12–15 U/kg Maximum total dose = 300 U[20,26]
OnabotulinumtoxinA (Botox)	100-U vial	12–16 U/kg (GMFCS V) Maximum total dose ≤300 U 16–20 U/kg (GMFCS I–IV) Maximum total dose ≤400–600 U[22]
RimabotulinumtoxinB (Myobloc)	2500 U in 0.5-mL vial 5000 U in 1-mL vial 10,000 U in 2-mL vial	No published dosing studies in children

Abbreviation: GMFCS, gross motor function classification system

aged 2 years and older, and the recommended dosing was based on a multicenter trial by Delgado and colleagues.[24] The equivalence ratio between ONA and ABO was suggested to be 1:3.[29] The use of conversion factors between different BoNT-A preparations is still strongly discouraged when switching from one drug to another because specific dosages are not interchangeable, reactions rates vary, and miscalculations may lead to life-threatening complications.[20,22]

There are currently no studies on rimabotulinumtoxinB dosing in children. A retrospective review of BoNT-B by Brandenburg and colleagues[30] with patients who were ONA nonresponders in their institution used doses ranging from 3000 to 22,000 U total (73.7–657.9 U/kg) and this was considered generally safe.

Contraindications to BoNT injection include hypersensitivity to any BoNT preparation and infection at the intended injection site. ABO in particular should not be used in patients with cow's milk protein allergy.[25] Injection frequency should be no less than 12-week intervals, and decision for retreatment based on clinical response, return of symptoms, and goals desired. The exact mechanism of the development of neutralizing antibody is unclear; however, increasing the interval between injections may decrease the prevalence of antibody production, which may be a contributing factor in cases of resistance manifested as inadequate or absent response to BoNT.[31,32] More importantly, in light of the known tendency for accelerated musculoskeletal aging and sarcopenia in individuals with CP, judicious use of BoNT should be exercised considering its possible contribution in furthering muscle atrophy and weakness. Multani and colleagues[33] recommend decreasing the frequency of administration to every 6 to 12 months and taking into account changes in muscle size, strength, and function with repeated injections.

All BoNT-A requires reconstitution with preservative-free 0.9% sodium chloride. The most effective dilution technique has not been established and is most often dictated by the number of muscles targeted and the volume needed to distribute the drug. Longer muscles may require 2 or more injection points, keeping a maximum of 50 U and/or 0.5 mL per site.[23]

PROCEDURE SETTING

The injection of BoNT can be administered with local or general anesthesia. Vibration, ice, and other distraction methods, including Child Life services, may be used in the outpatient setting to help ease the tension during the procedure. Muscle localization technique typically begins with simple manual palpation based on anatomic landmarks. A recent systematic review reveals strong evidence for more effective needle placement using instrumentation guidance with electromyography, electrical stimulation, and ultrasonography.[34]

ADVERSE EFFECTS

BoNT is generally considered safe. The most common adverse events reported are mild, localized reaction, which includes pain, swelling, and bruising at the site of injection and is often transient and self-limiting. On rare occasions, generalized weakness, fatigue, flulike symptoms, dry mouth, dysphagia, and breathing difficulty occur, suggestive of systemic and distant spread. There seem to be a higher risk of systemic adverse drug events in children than in adults, particularly those in GMFCS level IV and V, or those who have a history of dysphagia and/or aspiration pneumonia.[28] A pharmacoepidemiologic study of the World Health Organization VigiBase for adverse drug event reporting revealed an association between BoNT and death in children with CP.[35] Continued surveillance, accurate reporting, and further research are needed to better understand this complex relationship.[28]

CHEMONEUROLYSIS WITH PHENOL OR ALCOHOL

Phenol 5% to 7% and alcohol concentrations between 45% and 100% are proteolytic agents and, when injected in close proximity to a motor nerve, result in chemical neurolysis. They have the advantage of a rapid onset of action, longer duration of effect (up to 6–12 months), and lower cost. However, percutaneous injections typically require the use of electrical stimulation for localization, which may take up more time and require more skill to administer than toxins. The procedure can be painful and often requires the child to be sedated. There is a risk of painful dysesthesias when injected into a nerve with sensory fibers, muscle fibrosis, and scarring in surrounding tissues. Intravascular injection can cause systemic effects such as nausea, vomiting, muscle tremors, convulsions, depressed cardiac activity, blood pressure, and respiration.[36,37]

With the advent of ultrasonography visualization along with electrical stimulation, better localization is facilitated, thus reducing the volume of neurolytic agent needed to achieve clinical improvement.[38] Neurolysis in children with CP most often includes the obturator nerve for hip adductors, musculocutaneous nerve for the elbow flexor group, motor branch of the sciatic nerve supplying the hamstrings, and the medial popliteal nerve for spastic equinus. Dosing guidelines have not been established in children; however, 30 mg/kg has been thought to be safe.[36] In adults, single treatment sessions should not exceed 1 g (approximately 17 mL of 6% phenol).[39] Combining BoNT and phenol injection was noted to be safe, and allows more muscles to be treated while staying within the maximum dose for each.[40]

GENERAL PRINCIPLES AND SPECIAL CONSIDERATIONS IN SPASTICITY/HYPERTONIA MANAGEMENT IN CHILDREN WITH CEREBRAL PALSY

1. Distinguish presence and type of movement disorder, and how it influences function. A decision can be made on whether focal hypertonia management is indicated and which pharmacologic agent is most appropriate.
2. Identify muscles to be injected. Not all spastic muscles need to be treated, because some may rely on their hypertonia to maintain certain functions. It is also crucial to distinguish compensatory muscle activation (eg, intermittent toe flexion in standing to compensate for impaired balance). At times, there may be a need to purposefully weaken spastic muscles to allow for voluntary activation and strengthening. A single-event multilevel injection approach is often taken to maximize the treatment regimen, especially when both arms and legs are deemed to be needing treatment. The key-muscle concept by Strobl and colleagues[20] emphasizes the treatment goal being the next stage of physiologic motor development. **Fig. 1** shows this concept with suggested key muscles affected at each developmental stage.
3. Shared goals between the clinician and the patient/family. Outcome of treatment depend heavily on clear communication of goals for treatment. It is important that caregivers understand the expected effect of toxin injection, along with the need for other modalities in conjunction, such as strengthening and therapeutic exercise to achieve the motor function desired. Often, goals set are limited to addressing mainly body structure and function. A goal inventory list, as shown in **Fig. 2**, may help facilitate better discussion about goal setting between health care professionals and families, to also include activity and participation domains

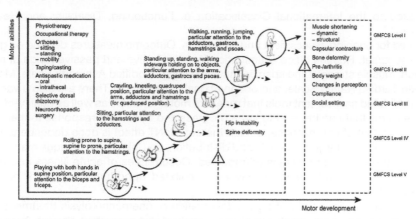

Fig. 1. Physiologic development/motor milestones with available therapy options listed in the left boxes. To every milestone, the affected muscles (key muscles for botulinum toxin injection) are shown. In cases of stagnation (*dashed arrows*), secondary alterations and deformities are shown in the right boxes. gastrocs, grastrocnemius. (*From* Strobl W, Theologis T, Brunner R, et al. Best clinical practice in botulinum toxin treatment for children with cerebral palsy. Toxins. 2015;7(5):1638.)

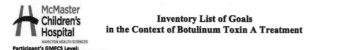

**Inventory List of Goals
in the Context of Botulinum Toxin A Treatment**

McMaster Children's Hospital
HAMILTON HEALTH SCIENCES

McMaster University
Department of Pediatrics

Participant's GMFCS Level: _____

Please read the following and mark the boxes beside the description that best represents the body structure and function, activity, and participation that you would like your child to achieve after botulinum toxin treatment.

I would like the botulinum toxin treatment to help my child to...

Body Structure / Function	Activity	Participation
Body Structure	□ Increase mobility	□ Be able to participate and compete
	□ and walk for longer distances	□ In wheelchair sports
Improve Range of Motion	□ and stand for longer periods of time	
□ In the legs	□ Facilitate ease of transfers in position (ex. from bed to	□ Recreational activities
□ and straighten the hips	chair) by care provider	□ Swimming
□ and straighten the knees		□ Biking
□ and straighten the ankle	□ Sit comfortably and with good posture	□ Community groups
□ In the arms	□ Be able to use assistive equipment	□ School activities
□ and raise the shoulders	□ and use a walker	
□ and straighten the elbows	□ and use a wheelchair	□ Religious activities
□ and straighten the wrists	□ and use a stander	
□ and bend and flex the fingers		
	□ Tolerate braces	
Function	□ and wear braces for a longer period of time	
□ Reduce overall muscle tone		
	□ Tolerate exercise	
□ Reduce the amount of drooling	□ and be able to do stretching exercises	
□ Reduce the feeling of generalized pain	□ Manipulate and use small objects with hands (e.g. writing supplies such as a pencil, light switches)	
□ Increase bone health and strengthen bones	□ Manage personal hygiene (e.g. diapering, toileting)	
	□ By patient	
□ Sleep with few disturbances	□ By care provider	
	□ Change clothes	
	□ and facilitate ease of dressing (e.g. socks, pants)	
	□ By patient	
	□ By care provider	
	□ and reduce the time taken to put on clothes	
	□ By patient	
	□ By care provider	
	□ Eat meals	
	□ and provide easier use of utensils	
	□ and reduce the time taken to eat meals	

Fig. 2. Goal inventory for botulinum toxin treatment. (*From* Nguyen L, Mesterman R, Gorter JW. Development of an inventory of goals using the International Classification of Functioning, Disability and Health in a population of nonambulatory children and adolescents with cerebral palsy treated with botulinum toxin A. BMC Pediatr. 2018;18:1.)

linked to the International Classification of Functioning, Disability and Health (ICF).[41]

4. Need for ongoing assessment and evaluation. Outcome measures depend on goal desired/set. Routine office examination includes active and passive range of motion, muscle strength and specific muscle testing, Modified Ashworth Scale, Modified Tardieu Rating Scale, and observational gait analysis. There are also a variety of validated assessment tools that measure motor function, as well as quality-of-life measures that can be used to track progress and document response to therapy.

5. Factors that affect response, or lack thereof. BoNT effect is dose dependent. Review of dosing, targeted muscle and distribution, and injection technique may show a need for these to be adjusted/modified. Occurrences of acute illness and pain can aggravate hypertonia or may have inhibited opportunities to work on the goal set.

6. Acknowledge limitations of chemodenervation or chemoneurolysis treatment. As children grow, their muscle structures and rheologic properties change. Younger children who used to benefit from BoNT injections to the gastrocnemius-soleus to decrease spastic equinus posture in walking may later develop fixed contractures and bony deformity that warrant surgical correction.

7. Rehabilitation therapy and other adjunct modalities. Given that motor disability is a hallmark of CP, physical and occupational therapies remain central in the management of such disorders. A rehabilitation program combining BoNT injections with physical therapy improved mobility, gait pattern, and muscle performance without increasing spasticity. Casting associated with BoNT improved range of motion and reduced spasticity better than BoNT alone. Data on electrical stimulation are inconclusive.[18,42]

DISCLOSURE

R. Dy has a research grant from IPSEN. D. Roge has nothing to disclose.

REFERENCES

1. Sanger TD, Delgado MR, Gaebler-Spira D, et al. Task Force on Childhood Motor Disorders. Classification and definition of disorders causing hypertonia in childhood. Pediatrics 2003;111:e89–97.

2. Jethwa A, Mink J, Macarthur C, et al. Development of the Hypertonia Assessment Tool (HAT): a discriminative tool for hypertonia in children. Dev Med Child Neurol 2010;52(5):e83–7.

3. Quality Standards Subcommittee of the American Academy of Neurology and the Practice Committee of the Child Neurology Society, Delgado MR, Hirtz D, Aisen M, et al. Practice parameter: pharmacologic treatment of spasticity in children and adolescents with cerebral palsy (an evidence-based review): report of the Quality Standards Subcommittee of the American Academy of Neurology and the Practice Committee of the Child. Neurology 2010;74(4):336–43.

4. Chang E, Ghosh N, Yanni D, et al. A review of spasticity treatments: pharmacological and interventional approaches. Crit Rev Phys Rehabil Med 2013;25(1–2): 11–22.

5. Chung CY, Chen CL, Wong AM. Pharmacotherapy of spasticity in children with cerebral palsy. J Formos Med Assoc 2011;110(4):215–22.

6. He Y, Brunstrom-Hernandez JE, Thio LL, et al. Population pharmacokinetics of oral baclofen in pediatric patients with cerebral palsy. J Pediatr 2014;164(5):1181–8.

7. Navarrete-Opazo AA, Gonzalez W, Nahuelhual P. Effectiveness of oral baclofen in the treatment of spasticity in children and adolescents with cerebral palsy. Arch Phys Med Rehabil 2016;97(4):604–18.
8. Lumsden DE, Kaminska M, Tomlin S, et al. Medication use in childhood dystonia. Eur J Paediatr Neurol 2016;20(4):625–9.
9. McLaughlin MJ, He Y, Brunstrom-Hernandez J, et al. Pharmacogenomic variability of oral baclofen clearance and clinical response in children with cerebral palsy. PM R 2018;10(3):235–43.
10. Fehlings D, Brown L, Harvey A, et al. Pharmacological and neurosurgical interventions for managing dystonia in cerebral palsy: a systematic review. Dev Med Child Neurol 2018;60(4):356–66.
11. Pozin I, Bdolah-Abram T, Ben-Pazi H. Levodopa does not improve function in individuals with dystonic cerebral palsy. J Child Neurol 2014;29:534–7.
12. Harvey A, Baker L, Reddihough D, et al. Trihexyphenidyl for dystonia in cerebral palsy. Cochrane Database Syst Rev 2018;(5):CD012430.
13. Liow NY, Gimeno H, Lumsden DE, et al. Gabapentin can significantly improve dystonia severity and quality of life in children. Eur J Paediatr Neurol 2016;20(1):100–7.
14. Carranza del Rio J, Clegg NJ, Moore A, et al. Use of trihexyphenidyl in children with cerebral palsy. Pediatr Neurol 2011;44:202–6.
15. Wong SS, Wilens TE. Medical cannabinoids in children and adolescents: a systematic review. Pediatrics 2017;140(5) [pii:e20171818].
16. Koppel BS, Brust JC, Fife T, et al. Systematic review: efficacy and safety of medical marijuana in selected neurologic disorders: report of the Guideline Development Subcommittee of the American Academy of Neurology. Neurology 2014; 82(17):1556–63.
17. Copeland K, Edwards P, Thorley M, et al. Botulinum toxin, A for nonambulatory children with cerebral palsy: a double blind randomized controlled trial. J Pediatr 2014;165(1):140–6.
18. Fonseca PR Jr, Calhes Franco de Moura R, Galli M, et al. Effect of physiotherapeutic intervention on the gait after the application of botulinum toxin in children with cerebral palsy: systematic review. Eur J Phys Rehabil Med 2018;54(5):757–65.
19. Graham HK, Rosenbaum P, Paneth N, et al. Cerebral palsy. Nat Rev Dis Primers 2016;2:15082.
20. Strobl W, Theologis T, Brunner R, et al. Best clinical practice in botulinum toxin treatment for children with cerebral palsy. Toxins (Basel) 2015;7(5):1629–48.
21. Hoare BJ, Wallen MA, Imms C, et al. Botulinum toxin A as an adjunct to treatment in the management of the upper limb in children with spastic cerebral palsy (UPDATE). Cochrane Database Syst Rev 2010;(1):CD003469.
22. Love SC, Novak I, Kentish M, et al, Cerebral Palsy Institute. Botulinum toxin assessment, intervention and after-care for lower limb spasticity in children with cerebral palsy: international consensus statement. Eur J Neurol 2010;17 Suppl 2:9–37.
23. Pavone V, Testa G, Restivo DA, et al. Botulinum toxin treatment for limb spasticity in childhood cerebral palsy. Front Pharmacol 2016;7:29.
24. Delgado MR, Tilton A, Russman B, et al. AbobotulinumtoxinA for equinus foot deformity in cerebral palsy: a randomized controlled trial. Pediatrics 2016; 137(2):e20152830.
25. Dysport (onabotulinumtoxinA) for Injection –FDA. Available at: https://www.accessdata.fda.gov/drugsatfda_docs/label/2016/125274s107lbl.pdf. Accessed March 24, 2019.

26. Carraro E, Trevisi E, Martinuzzi A. Safety profile of incobotulinum toxin A [Xeomin(®)] in gastrocnemious muscles injections in children with cerebral palsy: Randomized double-blind clinical trial. Eur J Paediatr Neurol 2016;20(4):532–7.
27. Koman LA, Mooney JF 3rd, Smith B, et al. Management of cerebral palsy with botulinum-A toxin: preliminary investigation. J Pediatr Orthop 1993;13(4):489–95.
28. Swinney CM, Bau K, Burton KLO, et al. Severity of cerebral palsy and likelihood of adverse events after botulinum toxin A injections. Dev Med Child Neurol 2018; 60(5):498–504.
29. Scaglione F. Conversion Ratio between Botox®, Dysport®, and Xeomin® in Clinical Practice. Toxins (Basel) 2016;8(3) [pii:E65].
30. Brandenburg JE, Krach LE, Gormley ME Jr. Use of rimabotulinum toxin for focal hypertonicity management in children with cerebral palsy with nonresponse to onabotulinum toxin. Am J Phys Med Rehabil 2013;92(10):898–904.
31. Oshima M, Deitiker P, Hastings-Ison T, et al. Antibody responses to botulinum neurotoxin type A of toxin-treated spastic equinus children with cerebral palsy: a randomized clinical trial comparing two injection schedules. J Neuroimmunol 2017;306:31–9.
32. Albrecht P, Jansen A, Lee JI, et al. High prevalence of neutralizing antibodies after long - term botulinum neurotoxin therapy. Neurology 2019;92(1):e48–54.
33. Multani I, Manji J, Tang MJ, et al. Sarcopenia, cerebral palsy, and botulinum toxin type A. JBJS Rev 2019;7(8):e4.
34. Grigoriu AI, Dinomais M, Rémy-Néris O, et al. Impact of injection-guiding techniques on the effectiveness of botulinum toxin for the treatment of focal spasticity and dystonia: a systematic review. Arch Phys Med Rehabil 2015;96(11):2067–78.
35. Montastruc J, Marque P, Moulis F, et al. Adverse drug reactions of botulinum neurotoxin type A in children with cerebral palsy: a pharmaco-epidemiological study in VigiBase. Dev Med Child Neurol 2017;59(3):329–34.
36. Gormley ME Jr, Krach LE, Piccini L. Spasticity management in the child with spastic quadriplegia. Eur J Neurol 2001;8(Suppl 5):127–35.
37. Elovic EP, Esquenazi A, Alter KE, et al. Chemodenervation and nerve blocks in the diagnosis and management of spasticity and muscle overactivity. PM R 2009;1(9):842–51.
38. Matsumoto ME, Berry J, Yung H, et al. Comparing electrical stimulation with and without ultrasound guidance for phenol neurolysis to the musculocutaneous nerve. PM R 2018;10(4):357–64.
39. Karri J, Mas MF, Francisco GE, et al. Practice patterns for spasticity management with phenol neurolysis. J Rehabil Med 2017;49(6):482–8.
40. Ploypetch T, Kwon JY, Armstrong HF, et al. A retrospective review of unintended effects after single-event multi-level chemoneurolysis with botulinum toxin-A and phenol in children with cerebral palsy. PM R 2015;7(10):1073–80.
41. Nguyen L, Mesterman R, Gorter JW. Development of an inventory of goals using the International Classification of Functioning, Disability and Health in a population of non-ambulatory children and adolescents with cerebral palsy treated with botulinum toxin A. BMC Pediatr 2018;18(1):1–10.
42. Mathevon L, Bonan I, Barnais JL, et al. Adjunct therapies to improve outcomes after botulinum toxin injection in children: A systematic review. Ann Phys Rehabil Med 2018;62(4):283–90.

Principles of Ankle-Foot Orthosis Prescription in Ambulatory Bilateral Cerebral Palsy

Ed Wright, MD[a],*, Sally A. DiBello, MPO, CPO[b,c]

KEYWORDS

- Cerebral palsy • Ankle-foot orthoses • Gait • AFO prescription

KEY POINTS

- Appropriate ankle-foot orthosis (AFO) prescription in ambulatory bilateral cerebral palsy (CP) is driven by the integrity of the plantar flexor–knee extension couple.
- Successful AFO prescription often requires interaction with complementary interventions.
- The angle of the ankle in the AFO must accommodate the knee-extended, midfoot-supported, dorsiflexion range of motion to optimize knee extension and midfoot integrity.
- AFO footwear modifications are necessary to reestablish normal gait function and alignment in AFOs designed to improve walking in CP.

 Video content accompanies this article at http://www.pmr.theclinics.com.

Ankle foot orthoses (AFOs) are the primary orthoses used to facilitate mobility in cerebral palsy (CP).[1] AFOs encompass the ankle joint and the whole or part of the foot, and are intended to control motion, correct deformity, and/or compensate for weakness.[2] AFOs vary widely by their design, materials, and stiffness. Changing any of these 3 components alters the effect the AFO has on gait.[3,4] For an AFO to improve gait function, it should promote normalization of the alignment of the ground reaction force (GRF) relative to the joints throughout the gait cycle (**Fig. 1**). Bringing the GRF closer to a joint reduces energy expenditure by the lower limb muscles (**Fig. 2**).[5]

For children with CP, alterations of lower extremity strength, tone, selectivity, motor coordination, and associated health conditions all have influence on their ambulatory progress. AFOs are prescribed to minimize the negative impact of these mechanical

[a] Texas Children's Hospital, 6701 Fannin Street, Suite 1280, Houston, TX 77030, USA; [b] Baylor College of Medicine School of Health Professions, One Baylor Plaza, MS: BCM115, Houston, TX 77030, USA; [c] Hanger Clinic, Houston, TX, USA
* Corresponding author.
E-mail address: exwrigh1@texaschildrens.org

Phys Med Rehabil Clin N Am 31 (2020) 69–89
https://doi.org/10.1016/j.pmr.2019.09.007
1047-9651/20/© 2019 Elsevier Inc. All rights reserved.

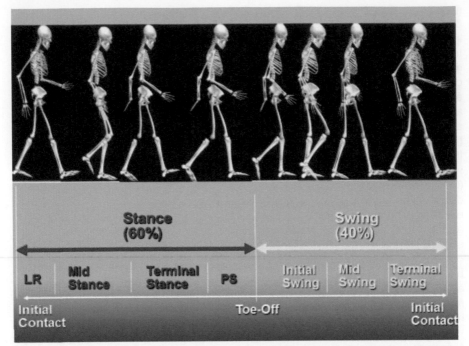

Fig. 1. The gait cycle begins and ends with the initial contact of 1 limb and is divided into stance and swing phases. LR, loading response; PS, preswing.

alterations by improving stability for walking, preserving range of motion (ROM), and moderating the deforming forces common to CP. AFOs are likely more effective at preventing, rather than alleviating, contractures and deformity in the foot and ankle.

Challenges exist to the "dosing" of orthoses (duration of wear and design) in ambulatory CP. One concern expressed is that restriction of motion in an orthosis

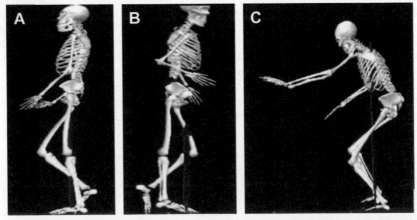

Fig. 2. The relationship of body weight to the GRF vector. (*A*) Optimal: GRF through the knee reduces muscle energy requirement. (*B*) GRF in front of the knee (recurvatum) disrupts forward momentum. (*C*) GRF behind the knee (crouch) increases antigravity muscle workload.

may inhibit the emergence of foot and ankle muscle use, limiting the development of typical movement patterns. For children with the mildest central nervous system injury, this concept may have merit. More consistently, impairments of motor control for selectivity and strength in distal musculature are a ceiling for the development of proper muscle function. Goal setting for an AFO, a critical element in prescribing, can create tensions between allowance of motion for functional goals and movement restriction to preserve musculoskeletal integrity. Some functional activities, such as transitioning to standing and stair climbing, benefit from more ankle ROM than is required for walking. Allowing for ankle dorsiflexion, as with a hinged AFO (HAFO), is based on this premise: that ankle motion is essential for the performance of normal movement patterns and postural responses.[6] However, when there is an ankle ROM limitation imposed by a tight gastrocsoleus complex (GSC), the allowance of dorsiflexion creates a circumstance favorable to breakdown of the midfoot. Compromise of midfoot integrity impairs postural response by weakening the foot lever, contributing to an unintended decline of posture in gait (crouch). Therefore, goals must be balanced. Consideration of strength, severity of spasticity, ankle ROM, and anticipation of potential for worsening crouch must factor into the decision rather than assuming that all children will benefit from 1 style of AFO rather than another. Introduction of an articulation also usually compromises intimacy of fit of the brace and control of the hindfoot may be lost. Increased mediolateral motion may increase and skin issues may result.

Research shows that AFOs affect a variety of gait parameters; however, reported outcomes are not all in agreement. There is wide variability in the existing CP/orthotic outcomes research. Inadequacy in the descriptions of participants (tone, Gross Motor Function Classification System [GMFCS], ROM, gait type), AFO details (type, motion, materials, goals), and testing protocols (controls, randomization, acclimation) are cited to account for this.[7]

A recent systematic review of posterior AFOs in ambulatory CP offers an overview of the studied impacts of posterior AFOs (this review had limited data for the use floor reaction AFOs [FR-AFOs]). Pooled data revealed strong evidence for benefit to temporal spatial parameters, stride length more than cadence more than gait speed, and moderate evidence for improvements in gross motor function as measured by relevant subsets of the Gross Motor Function Measure and Pediatric Evaluation of Disability Inventory. There was limited, nonsupportive evidence of impact on balance, activities of daily living, stair climbing, activity level, or energy costs. Improved ankle kinematics for equinus gait in stance and swing were noted, but there was no reported change in knee and hip kinematics. Gait parameters improved in unilateral CP to a greater degree than bilateral CP.[8] Orthoses with trim lines that encompass only the foot, such as the University of California Biomechanics Laboratory (UCBL) and supramalleolar orthoses (SMOs) may have some benefit to bony deformity risks; however, they do not have measurable impact on gait.[9]

NORMAL MOTION AND FUNCTION OF THE FOOT DURING GAIT

Readers less familiar with hindfoot and midfoot anatomy and motion are referred to https://www.youtube.com/watch?v=0R4zRSE_-40 4:52-5:15 & 5:52-6:57.

Successful AFO management in ambulatory bilateral CP requires a foundational understanding of the typical function of the ankle and foot during the gait cycle. The subtalar joint constitutes the articulation between the talus and calcaneus (**Fig. 3**). It acts synergistically with the midfoot and ankle joints in all 3 planes of motion with

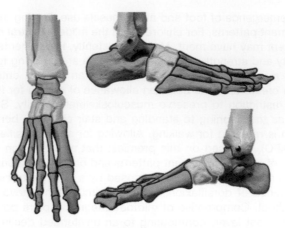

Fig. 3. Typical anatomy of the hindfoot (*blue*), midfoot (*green*), and forefoot (*purple*).

an axis nearly 45° out of both the axial and coronal planes (**Fig. 4**A). Subtalar motion is comparable with a miter gear, converting internal and external rotation of leg into pronation and supination of the foot respectively (**Fig. 4**B).

Our limbs cycle through these motions (**Fig. 5**) across the gait cycle. A pronated foot is supple and ideal for both shock absorption and adaptation to variations in terrain needed during weight acceptance (loading response). A supinated foot is rigid, serving as a strong lever arm for the calf musculature to exert the force required to propel the limb forward at push-off. When the foot initially comes into full contact with the floor, the leg internally rotates maximally, and the foot pronates. Pronation occurs primarily through the subtalar joint by eversion of the calcaneus. Calcaneal eversion allows the talus to adduct and plantar flex, which unlocks the midfoot as the talonavicular and calcaneocuboid joints gain a parallel or convergent axis (**Fig. 6**).

As soon as body weight is fully transferred to the outstretched stance limb, it begins to externally rotate as the pelvis and swing limb rotate forward. External rotation of the limb lifts the talus into a dorsiflexed and abducted position, allowing inversion of the calcaneus. The axes of the talonavicular and calcaneocuboid joints become progressively divergent and the flexibility of the foot declines.

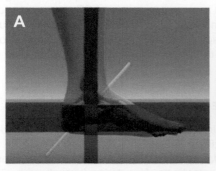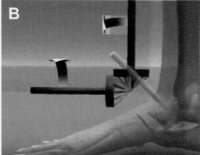

Fig. 4. (*A*) Axis of the subtalar joint. (*B*). Relationship of shank rotation and foot motion. (*Courtesy of* [*B*] Dr. Glass DPM; available at https://www.youtube.com/watch?v=0R4zRSE_-40; with permission.)

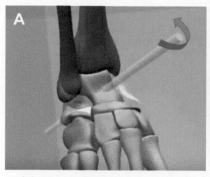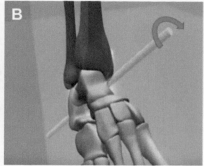

Fig. 5. (*A*) Leg internal rotation coupled to foot pronation. (*B*) Leg external rotation coupled to foot supination.

The ability of the foot to become a progressively rigid lever is critical to stability in midstance and torque production by the plantar flexors during terminal stance (**Fig. 7**).

THE PLANTAR FLEXOR–KNEE EXTENSION COUPLE

The soleus restrains excessive motion of the tibia (shank) as the ankle dorsiflexes during midstance (second rocker). The impact of the restrained shank on knee stability during the second rocker is known as the plantar flexor–knee extension couple (PF-KE). The effectiveness of the PF-KE in CP depends on 3 elements.

1. Function of the plantar flexors: strength, timing, tone, and length
2. Structural integrity of the bones and ligaments of the foot (lever arm integrity)
3. Direction of foot progression during walking (foot progression angle)

When any of these elements are disrupted, the function of the plantar flexors to act as knee stabilizers is compromised. The child may have to rely on energy-inefficient patterns of muscle activity, such as continuous quadriceps activity in stance, to maintain knee extension (see **Fig. 2**C).

Children's body mass, proximal tone, contractures, and strength influence the force requirement of the PF-KE and thus its effectiveness. In that sense a stabilizing orthosis

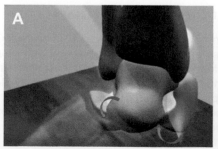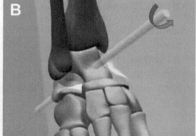

Fig. 6. (*A*) Subtalar pronation: talus plantar flexion and adduction with calcaneal eversion. (*B*) Foot pronation: midfoot arch is flattened (unlocked) and the midfoot and forefoot can dorsiflexion and abduct.

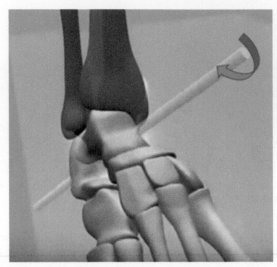

Fig. 7. Foot supination: midfoot arch narrows and peaks (locks), restricting midfoot and forefoot motion.

that works from the bottom up may be overwhelmed by top-down impairments. As such, orthopedic referral to improve ankle ROM, restore foot integrity, and address proximal deformities is often necessary for an AFO to provide benefit to more involved children.

FOOT AND LEG DEFORMITIES AND DEVIATIONS OF THE PLANTAR FLEXOR–KNEE EXTENSION

Children with CP often develop foot deformities that disrupt the normal pattern of subtalar joint motion and the benefits thereof. Three foot and ankle malalignments are common in CP.[9] Equinus and equinoplanovalgus are common in bilateral CP. Equinus is the result of fixed or dynamic GSC shortening, resulting in calcaneal plantar flexion. This condition creates an excessive PF-KE (see **Fig. 2**B). Equinus in bilateral CP commonly gives way to equinoplanovalgus with calcaneal plantar flexion/eversion and associated excessive midfoot pronation. This midfoot compromise results in substantial weakening of the PF-KE (see **Fig. 2**C).

EQUINOPLANOVALGUS: MIDFOOT BREAKDOWN IN BILATERAL CEREBRAL PALSY

Equinoplanovalgus foot deformity is common, although not universal, in bilateral CP. Equinoplanovalgus is problematic because although calcaneal eversion with pronation of the subtalar joint is normal during loading response, the foot must sufficiently recover to a supinated position to respond to plantar flexor force effectively. Failure to supinate adequately limits the development of the foot rigidity necessary for an effective PF-KE. This inadequacy becomes further amplified during terminal stance when propulsive force generation is required. The propulsive force of the gastrocsoleus on a supple, pronated foot stresses the ligamentous and bony structures of the medial midfoot, which elongate and deform over time.

Several forces favor the persistent foot pronation that eventually progresses to the equinoplanovalgus foot.

- Children with bilateral CP are typically transitioning to weight bearing between 18 and 60 months, when pronation of the foot is physiologic.[10]
- Internal rotation of the lower limb as a result of persistent femoral anteversion.
- A tight GSC acts to both limit ankle dorsiflexion and hold the calcaneus in a plantar flexed and everted position. During second rocker the dorsiflexion becomes a shared motion between the ankle and the foot as GSC tethering of ankle dorsiflexion forces this motion to occur in the midfoot. A so-called second or little ankle develops as the midfoot become excessively dorsiflexed and abducted (equinoplanovalgus) (**Fig. 8**).

This condition is a good example of bony deformities in need of orthopedic evaluation before orthotic intervention. Commonly, as weight bearing progresses and the foot lever fails, the internally rotated femur and abducted forefoot generates a torque on the tibia that promotes external torsion of this bony segment. The combination of heel equinus, talonavicular subluxation, midfoot break, and external tibial torsion contributes to lever arm dysfunction commonly associated with crouch[11] (**Fig. 9**).

GROWTH AND STAGES IN BILATERAL CEREBRAL PALSY GAIT

Activity levels, tone, strength, deformity, and body mass all affect changes in the gait patterns of children with bilateral CP. Graham and Rodda[12] characterized these gait patterns and offered treatment schemata for each. Although this is not a strict continuum in bilateral CP, it helps clinicians to understand the key components for an orthotic prescription.

Early walking for children with bilateral CP is characterized by a plantar flexed ankle position caused by GSC shortening. Frequently this more dynamic than static and proximal tone is often limited. In these, usually smaller, children there is ample integrity of the foot relative to body mass, so that the PF-KE is strong, promoting knee extension during all phases of stance. This early stage is referred to as toe walking or equinus gait (**Fig. 10**A). When there is more significant proximal muscle tone, shortening, or weakness, as occurs with growth and weight gain, the result is increased hip and knee flexion during stance. In time, the integrity of the foot lever begins to compromise and the PF-KE with it. As the stance limb accepts the full weight of the body, the knees and hips become biased toward flexion. This stage characterizes jump gait, and knee and hip extension are incomplete during stance (**Fig.10**B, C). These 2 gait patterns are common to GMFCS levels I to III.

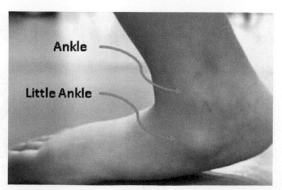

Fig. 8. Little ankle. Dorsiflexion occurs through the midfoot joints rather than the true ankle joint.

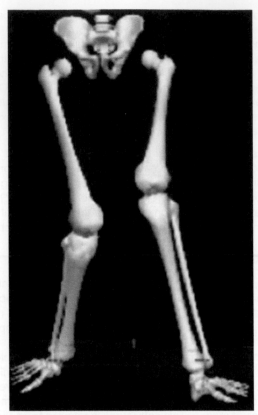

Fig. 9. Talonavicular subluxation, midfoot breakdown, and external tibial torsion contributing to lever arm dysfunction during crouch gait.

With progression of proximal tone and weakness, and lever arm dysfunction at the foot and tibia, the PF-KE couple weakens further and apparent equinus develops (**Fig. 10**D). Toe walking at this stage is reflective of flexion at the knee and hip flexion, rather than true plantar flexion of the ankle and foot. This position can occur as the

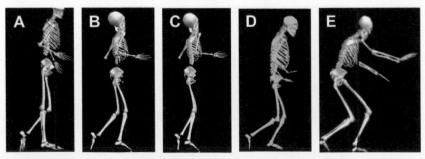

Fig. 10. (*A*) Equinus: ankle plantar flexed, knee and hip extended (Video 1). (*B, C*) Jump gait: ankle plantar flexed, knee and hip flex then jump back into incomplete extension (Video 2). (*D*) Apparent equinus: toe walking reflects knee and hip flexion (Video 3). (*E*) Crouch: ankle dorsiflexion, knee and hip flexion (Video 4).

natural history in bilateral CP, with a plantar flexed calcaneus and midfoot dorsiflexion but is also frequently seen when GSC release allows calcaneal dorsiflexion. Finally, the fully compromised PF-KE, with foot and ankle dorsiflexion, proximal flexion contractures, and worsening muscle strength to body mass ratio, leads to crouch gait, with severe knee and hip flexion (**Fig. 10**E). This gait pattern is nonsustainable or declining through adulthood. These last 2 gait types commonly function at GMFCS III to IV.

The major goal of orthotic management in bilateral CP is, from the bottom up, to dampen the progressive compromise of the PF-KE couple in stance; the product of proximal tone, relative strength decline, and progressive lever arm dysfunction. This goal may be beyond the capacity of an orthosis to manage and appropriate top-down complementary interventions must be pursued.

NAMING CONVENTIONS AND BASIC MATERIALS SCIENCE FOR LOWER LIMB ORTHOSES

Orthoses are named by the joints they cross; for example, an AFO is an orthosis that encompasses the ankle and foot. A knee AFO is an orthosis that encompasses the knee, ankle, and foot. This naming convention applies to upper or lower limb orthoses, and spinal orthoses. Orthoses are thought to provide direct control to the joints they encompass and provide indirect control of the next joint proximal. For example, an AFO provides direct control over the ankle and indirect control over the knee. It is possible to increase or decrease the effect an AFO has on knee motion by adjusting the amount of control over the ankle joint. The amount of influence is achieved through the materials selected, the trim lines of the orthosis, and various types of mechanical ankle components (eg, joints, straps) available.

A few of the most common materials used for custom AFOs are copolymer, polypropylene, and polyethylene plastics. Plastics offer the advantages of custom molding, creating an intimate contact with the foot and ankle of the wearer. Some plastics are very flexible, and some are more rigid. These different types of plastics are chosen based on the goals of the orthosis. If the goal of the AFO is to restrict motion or increase support to the leg, a more rigid plastic can be used; if the goal of the AFO is to allow greater joint motion, more flexible plastics can be used. Off-the-shelf carbon fiber products offer a lighter-weight alternative to plastics and may offer some measure of energy storage/return. A carbon fiber AFO can often interface with a custom-molded plastic supramalleolar AFO to achieve more intimate contact.

Orthotic trim lines delineate how much of the limb is encompassed by the plastic material and affect the amount of control or support provided to the user. For example, the trim lines of a typical solid-ankle AFO (SAFO) cross the ankle at the apices of the malleoli, whereas the trim lines of a typical posterior leaf spring AFO cross the ankle posterior to the apices of the malleoli. Because there is less plastic surrounding the ankle to resist motion during ambulation, the posterior leaf spring AFO allows more dorsiflexion ROM during stance than the SAFO. In a similar manner, the amount of support provided can be modified by changing the amount of plastic on the bottom of the foot, or the foot plate. The shorter the foot plate, the less supportive the orthosis. Trim lines can be considered another feature of the AFO that should be customized to suit the needs of each patient.

Similarly, various mechanical ankle components can be used to limit or encourage motion at the ankle. It is helpful to think of these mechanical components in relation to their function. Some joints, such as the Tamarack joint (**Fig. 11**), have viscoelastic properties that provide assistance into dorsiflexion. Other components, such as the dorsiflexion restraint strap, can provide dorsiflexion restraint, or stop it entirely, in smaller patients. The range of lower limb orthotic componentry continues to expand

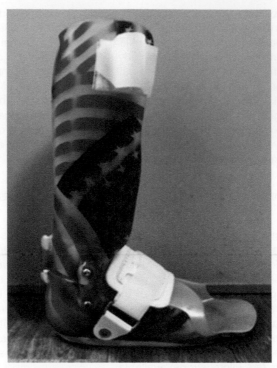

Fig. 11. A HAFO with free dorsiflexion ROM and a plantar flexion stop set at 90°. Optimal use requires true ankle dorsiflexion ROM and an intact PF-KE couple.

with technological advances. More componentry options and advanced technologies are discussed later in this article.

ORTHOTIC MANAGEMENT OF GAIT DYSFUNCTION IN BILATERAL CEREBRAL PALSY

When the goal of an AFO is to promote ambulation, the appropriate orthotic prescription, regardless of the age or GMFCS level of the child, requires the clinician to perform a thorough physical examination and observational gait analysis. Identifying the gait type is useful in guiding orthotic options. Appropriate strengthening, tone reduction, and orthopedic interventions should be promoted. Lower-limb orthoses function optimally when designed based on sound biomechanical reasoning and when used in conjunction with complementary interventions (**Fig. 12**).

EQUINUS GAIT

Children with equinus gait typically present with excessive knee extension (excessive PF-KE couple). Although these children may appear to achieve a flat foot during mid-stance, physical examination commonly reveals hypertonicity of the plantar flexors and limited ankle dorsiflexion ROM. It should be appreciated that children often achieve this flat foot posture by stealing ROM from the knee joint or the foot, resulting in undesirable compensations of recurvatum at the knee or dorsiflexion of the midfoot. Unless the hypertonicity and limited ankle ROM are addressed or considered within the orthotic design, the orthosis will be ineffective in improving gait function. Therefore, orthotic treatment goals for this gait type depend on the severity of GSC

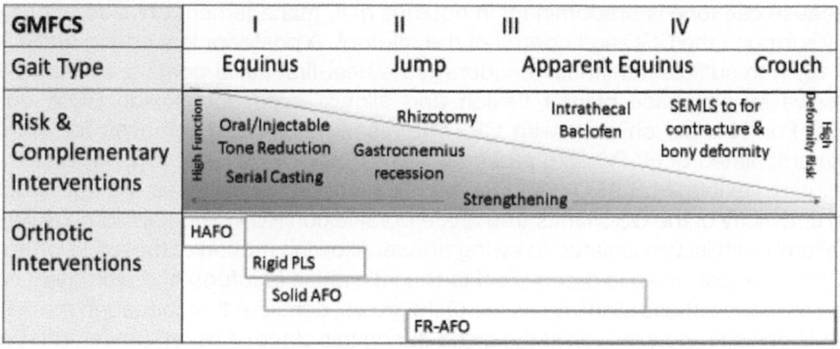

GMFCS	I		II	III		IV	
Gait Type	Equinus		Jump	Apparent Equinus		Crouch	
Risk & Complementary Interventions	High Function	Oral/Injectable Tone Reduction Serial Casting	Rhizotomy Gastrocnemius recession Strengthening		Intrathecal Baclofen	SEMLS to for contracture & bony deformity	High Deformity Risk
Orthotic Interventions	HAFO						
		Rigid PLS					
			Solid AFO				
				FR-AFO			

Fig. 12. The general relationship between GMFCS level and gait dysfunction in CP. As deformity risk increases and function decreases, interventions are often more involved. PLS, posterior leaf spring; SEMLS, single-event multilevel surgery.

shortening and the effectiveness of complementary interventions in restoring ankle dorsiflexion. If adequate gastrocnemius length is achieved, the orthosis can allow dorsiflexion during stance and activities such as stair climbing and transition from floor to standing.

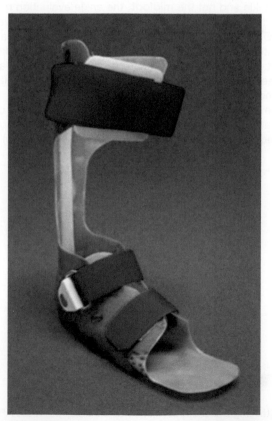

Fig. 13. A custom-molded thermoplastic PLS AFO with posterior reinforcement to increase stiffness as needed. Provides minimal second rocker support, promotes swing clearance while supporting mild foot deformity.

Because calf tone is predominant in equinus gait, management considerations primarily surround the GSC and control of the midfoot. A posterior leaf spring (PLS) AFO (**Fig. 13**) with sufficient stiffness encourages a heel-first initial contact by controlling excessive swing phase plantar flexion and allows ankle dorsiflexion ROM during stance. For younger children with CP, commonly prescribed orthoses for equinus are an articulated or HAFO with a plantar flexion stop at 90° (see **Fig. 11**) or a traditional, very flexible, PLS AFO (see **Fig. 13**). These types of orthoses are not effective when spasticity of the GSC limits true ankle dorsiflexion ROM and should be reserved for children with issues isolated to swing phase. Allowing motion at the ankle when the GSC range is restrained is detrimental to the little ankle (midfoot) and ultimately compromises stance phase stability. As the child grows, consider that, although more flexible AFO designs allow motion at the ankle during this stage of development, this same motion may be detrimental to stance phase stability as spasticity increases and more severe gait deviations develop.

EQUINUS GAIT WITH RECURVATUM

Children who have been less responsive to efforts at restoring gastrocnemius ROM often present with a degree of equinus associated with recurvatum. AFO design must accommodate this ROM limitation. To ensure the child's dorsiflexion ROM is coming from the ankle and not the midfoot, the ankle evaluation must be done with the knee extended and the midfoot bias toward supination/heel varus because full knee extension ROM is required for normal gait function. If clinicians seek to reestablish normal gait patterns, the give-and-take nature of the ankle and knee joint must be understood. Most children with CP achieve a greater degree of ankle dorsiflexion ROM with the knee flexed, rather than extended, which should be taken into consideration during orthotic design decision making.

Difficulties achieving a successful orthotic intervention for these children are often related to a mismatch of the patient's knee-extended, midfoot-supported, ankle dorsiflexion ROM and the angle of the ankle in the AFO (AA-AFO) (**Fig. 14**). If, on

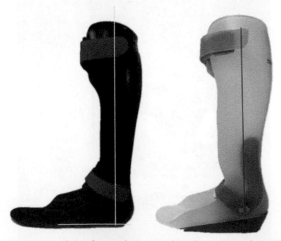

Fig. 14. AA-AFO is the angle of the foot relative to the tibia within the AFO. The AFO on the right shows a plantar flexed AA-AFO with in-the-shoe wedging on the plantar surface to accommodate the contracture present. The AFO on the left shows a plantigrade/90° AA-AFO.

examination, neutral dorsiflexion is not available at the true ankle (ie, knee flexion or midfoot dorsiflexion is substituted for true ankle dorsiflexion) and an AFO is set at 90°, the structural stability of the midfoot is lost and the orthosis can contribute to progressive lever arm dysfunction, discomfort, skin breakdown, and potential abandonment of the orthosis. In addition, because of the interactive nature of ankle and knee joint ROM, it is likely that the AFO will not effectively address gait deviations occurring at the knee. Therefore, it is the knee-extended, midfoot-supported, ankle dorsiflexion ROM that determines the AA-AFO. Understanding the synergistic nature of the midfoot, ankle, and knee joints allows clinicians to identify children whose range limitation is such that surgical intervention is an appropriate consideration before AFO prescription. If a knee-extended ankle plantar flexion contracture greater than 10° exists, AFO accommodations inside the shoe can become a barrier to successful use of the orthosis.

Because of the aforementioned risks of misidentifying ankle dorsiflexion ROM in children with equinus gait who show recurvatum, a PLS or HAFO is likely unsuitable. Gait abnormalities in these children are best managed with an SAFO (**Fig. 15**). SAFOs are designed to prevent ankle dorsiflexion and plantar flexion during stance phase and, in doing so, provide indirect support to, or control of, the knee joint. Because the SAFO encompasses a greater surface area of the lower limb, it is also indicated when there is a need to control undesired triplanar deformity of the midfoot.

When the gastrocnemius does not have sufficient length to allow ankle dorsiflexion during stance, children maintain forward progression of their bodies by stealing

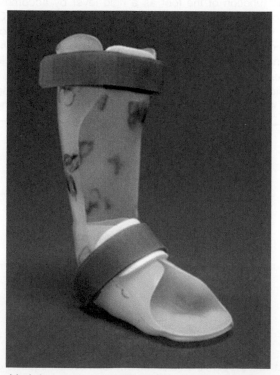

Fig. 15. Custom-molded thermoplastic SAFO. Designed to provide triplanar control of foot and ankle deformities and improve control of the knee joint during ambulation. Can be used with or without the inner boot seen here.

motion from the midfoot (breakdown) or knee (recurvatum). This concept still holds true if it is the AFO that is limiting ankle dorsiflexion ROM (rather than a physiologic contracture). Because available passive ankle dorsiflexion ROM is a major contributor to recurvatum during stance phase,[13,14] the AA-AFO must sufficiently accommodate the plantar flexion contracture of the AFO-footwear combination (AFO-FC) to encourage appropriate knee extension (**Fig. 16**). The position of the ankle within the AFO is a key determining factor in the ability of the AFO in controlling recurvatum. In order to accomplish this, the SAFO should accommodate the plantar flexion contracture through use of wedging material. Appropriate shoe wear to place the lower limb in proper alignment adds further control (discussed later). Accommodation of the ankle plantar flexion contracture also improves control of the midfoot within the orthosis, which prevents skin callusing and discomfort during weight bearing. An AFO can be used to limit midfoot breakdown through strong soft tissue support under the subtalar joint, but only if the contracture is first accommodated.

JUMP GAIT

Jump gait is characterized by ankle plantar flexion in stance with excessive flexion of the knees and hips. The PF-KE is insufficient to fully extend these proximal joints against stiff and weak proximal muscles. Complementary treatments are focused on proximal tone reduction and strengthening. Correction of ankle and foot deformity and stabilization of the ankle in the sagittal plane should be prioritized over allowing ankle motion at this stage. Orthotic management of jump gait must be focused on reestablishing the function of the foot as a rigid lever by accommodating existing gastrocnemius contracture and supporting the midfoot within the AFO. This focus optimizes the ability of the orthosis to support appropriate knee extension during stance. If properly aligned, the AFO can facilitate larger step length, which can encourage normal lengthening of the hip flexors and the GSC, potentially enhancing the therapeutic effects of spasticity management.

For smaller children with mild amounts of knee and hip flexion during ambulation, an SAFO that is stiff enough to support the weight of the body during single-limb support

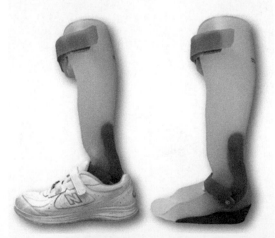

Fig. 16. The effect that proper AFO-FC alignment can have on equinus gait with recurvatum. The AA-AFO must match the child's ankle ROM limitations. The wedging under the AFO in combination with the effective shoe heel height create an alignment favorable to correction of recurvatum.

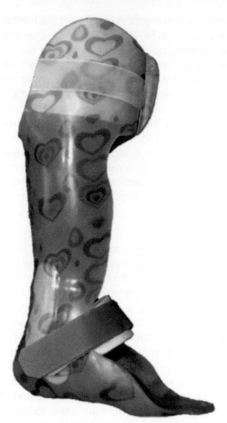

Fig. 17. A custom-molded thermoplastic FR-AFO. Also known as a ground reaction AFO. This AFO more effectively increases knee extension by replacing the proximal anterior strap with a rigid anterior panel.

is most appropriate. As the degree of stance phase knee flexion becomes more severe with increasing body mass, an FR-AFO (or ground reaction AFO) may provide greater support at the knee (**Fig. 17**). The rigid anterior panel helps resist excessive knee flexion by acting synergistically with the rigid toe plate of the FR-AFO. As with any AFO design, accommodation of existing ankle contracture and proper realignment of the lower limb in the coronal and transverse planes is key to management of stance phase deviations at the knee.

APPARENT EQUINUS

Because of the growing influence of proximal impairments, complementary interventions must be multilevel, often involving systemic tone reduction and orthopedics to effect a more upright posture. The AFO must ensure that midfoot stability is maintained. Allowing midfoot dorsiflexion in order to keep the foot plantigrade is undesirable in this population because it represents a failure of the foot as a rigid lever for the GSC to act on and can be expected to worsen over time. For smaller, higher-functioning children who present with apparent equinus and lesser amounts of hip and knee flexion, an SAFO with appropriate stiffness, alignment, and accompanying footwear effectively increases stance phase knee extension. Commonly, an FR-AFO is necessary to accomplish this.

Either of these AFO designs can function to support the midfoot, improve alignment of the lower limb, and enhance the PF-KE couple as long as the angle of the ankle in the AFO accommodates existing contractures. A plantar flexed angle of the ankle in the AFO in this population mitigates some of the negative effects of a spastic or contracted GSC and improves control of the midfoot by creating less tension on both the midfoot and the knee joint. Relaxing the GSC at the ankle improves the ability of the AFO to increase knee extension, because of the biarticular nature of the gastrocnemius. Slight plantar flexion within the AFO also resists midfoot compromise. A full-length toe plate increases the length of the mechanical lever arm of the orthosis, increasing resistance to knee flexion in stance. The effectiveness of the FR-AFO in improving knee extension depends on successful attention to proximal muscle impairments. FR-AFOs in isolation (without medical or surgical management of the proximal segments) in this population can result in suboptimal management of gait dysfunction.

CROUCH GAIT

When the PF-KE couple becomes fully compromised, the result is crouch gait. This gait is characterized by excessive foot and ankle dorsiflexion with severe knee and hip flexion and is frequently associated with rotational deformity. This gait pattern presents a major challenge to successful orthotic intervention. Children with crouch gait who present with slow walking velocity, weak plantar flexors, and an externally rotated foot progression angle were found to benefit the most from bilateral FR-AFO intervention.[15] Other investigators have considered greater than 15° of external tibia rotation a contraindication.[16] The primary goal for AFOs for children with crouch gait is to reestablish the PF-KE couple, increase knee extension, improve step length, and improve gait speed. Commonly, multilevel orthopedic interventions are also being considered for this population. Proximal limitations of hip and knee flexion ROM and external foot progression angle related to tibial torsion may need to be addressed to provide maximal benefit.

Selecting the appropriate angle of the ankle in the AFO remains key to successful orthotic management of crouch gait. It is the most predictive factor in determining how much improvement in knee extension can be expected from an AFO used to treat excessive knee flexion.[17] Effectiveness also depends on the stiffness of the orthosis in combination with the shoe and the alignment of the AFO. Although limited, there is evidence that AFOs used after single-event multilevel surgery (SEMLS) provide greater improvements in gait parameters than SEMLS alone,[18] supporting the idea that surgical and orthotic intervention both play important roles in achieving a more upright posture.

ANKLE FOOT ORTHOSIS TUNING CONCEPTS

Commonly, an AFO is designed in isolation, meaning that little consideration is given to the effect that footwear can have on the overall effectiveness of the orthosis. The notion that footwear must be considered as an integral part of the orthotic prescription for ambulatory children with CP was brought to the mainstream by Elaine Owen[19] MBE, MSc, SRP, MCSP. This approach prioritizes realignment of the shank (or tibia) and the thigh to encourage normal motion of these segments throughout each phase of gait. Foundational to successful AFO intervention is the concept that realignment of the shank into a normal position (10° inclined) is possible, even for children with limited ankle ROM, because the AFO-FC can recreate this normalized position. **Fig. 18** shows a child with an angle of the ankle in the AFO set at 7° plantar flexion with modifications done to the footwear that realign the shank to a position of 10° inclined to vertical.

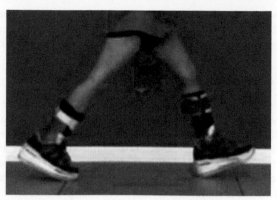

Fig. 18. The beneficial effects of proper AFO-FC tuning. AA-AFO set at 5° plantar flexed to accommodate contractures and maintain good alignment of the midfoot. Heel wedging inside the shoe to accommodate contracture and shoe modifications realign the shank to a normal position. Shoe modifications increase knee extension to create big V. Big V may assist in maintaining normal length of hip flexors and gastrocnemius.

Reestablishing the inclined position of the shank during stance phase mimics the position of the lower limb typically created by normal ankle dorsiflexion ROM and ankle stiffness that many children with CP are lacking. Additional benefits include more normal alignment of the center of mass over the base of the foot and anterior to the knee.

Children who benefit the most from this approach are those lacking ankle dorsiflexion ROM and who therefore require an SAFO. The potential drawbacks to a design that restricts motion at the ankle can be addressed through modifications to the AFO-FC. The SAFO provides necessary stability to the ankle and knee during midstance because of its restriction of ankle dorsiflexion; however, the entrance to midstance (initial contact and loading response) and exit from midstance (terminal stance) must be optimized by modification of the shoe sole. This modification is accomplished by changing the profile of the heel and the forefoot of the shoe (see **Fig. 18**). Modification of the heel profile can speed up or slow down the rate at which the foot becomes flat on the floor, allowing the clinician to provide more or less stability to the knee during loading response. The forefoot profile determines the exit from midstance, meaning it establishes the amount and timing of knee stability through terminal stance. Modification of the forefoot profile is ideally done with a point-loading rocker. These sole modifications require increased sole height. Sole heights can effectively accommodate ankle PF contractures up to 10° before the sole height limits the utility of this approach. Contractures of greater magnitude likely require surgical consideration.

The amount of shank inclination and the heel and sole profile of the AFO-FC are optimized using video gait analysis and GRF data to go through a process called tuning. Tuning refers to the process of making small adjustments in order to optimize the function of the AFO-FC for a specific activity, most commonly walking. Ideally, prescription of an AFO-FC for children with CP includes a high degree of collaboration between the physician, physical therapist, family, and orthotist. The use of the word tuning is widespread among orthotists in the United States, although only a handful of clinical groups are fully engaging in this process as it was originally intended. Perhaps one of the most important results of Owen's[19] efforts in the United States is the enhanced focus on alignment principles for lower limb orthotics in general. Repositioning of the shank and thigh and consideration of the effect of the footwear on the function of the

AFO have become more common since the introduction of this approach, regardless of the type of AFO used. The changes brought about by exposure to this treatment philosophy have without a doubt improved the standard of care for children with CP.

MATERIALS AND COMPONENTRY FOR LOWER LIMB ORTHOSES

The amount of support provided by an orthosis is heavily influenced by the materials and componentry available. AFO fabrication has traditionally been completed using various types of heat-moldable plastics, or thermoplastics, as mentioned previously. In general, thermoplastic AFOs allow small changes to be made to accommodate the child's growth. Custom-molded AFOs, which are molded intimately to the children's anatomy, allow small changes to be made as they grow. This intimate fit can be ideal to meet specific treatment goals. Prescribing providers should recognize that off-the-shelf or custom-fit thermoplastic AFOs are fabricated from size charts that are not custom molded, which can compromise the necessary intimacy of fit and loss of control of deformity or support.

Recent advances in the materials and componentry available have increased the orthotic design options significantly. AFOs made of carbon fiber behave differently than AFOs made of other materials because of the properties of the material. Depending on the specific design, carbon fiber AFOs can provide energy storage and return, which means that energy is stored in the AFO as the ankle dorsiflexes during a step, and energy is returned as the AFO is unloaded. This concept is commonly referred to as dynamic response and is thought to mimic the typical function of the ankle muscles during walking more closely than thermoplastics. Carbon fiber AFOs such as the Kiddie Gait from Allard USA, and a multitude of others, provide dynamic response and are appropriate for children with mild strength deficits, mild foot deformities, and who have successful tone management in place. Because these off-the-shelf carbon fiber AFOs are sized based on the child's foot length, they can be limited in the range of children they are appropriate for but are advantageous because they are cost-effective and lightweight. They can also interface with UCBLs or SMOs if a greater measure of foot support is required.

For children with CP who are older or have more severe deficits in their gait patterns or muscle strength, carbon fiber AFOs can be custom molded. Creating a custom carbon fiber AFO allows the orthotist to fully customize the amount of support provided by the orthosis. Custom-molded carbon AFOs provide an intimate fit, improved control of deformity, and increased comfort along with energy storage and return. These types of AFOs are more costly and some designs are unable to be modified significantly to accommodate a child's growth. Therefore, use of custom-molded carbon fiber AFOs should likely be limited to the most severe cases, or for older children with CP whose growth has slowed.

Other design advances for AFOs include new ankle joints that provide a wider range of support and adjustability for children who have changing needs. Many of these ankle joints feature an anterior and/or posterior channel that provides individual assistance to weak dorsiflexors or plantar flexors. Others block motion in 1 direction but allow movement in the other direction. This property allows fine-tuned adjustments to the amount of support or ROM provided by the AFO, should the patient's goals or physical capacity change while using the orthosis. Added orthotic bulk is a disadvantage of using mechanical ankle joints.

Although advances in materials and componentry have increased the options for orthotic design, it is important to keep in mind that these advances cannot typically

Table 1			
A summary of gait pattern, recommended orthotic intervention, and considerations			
Gait Pattern	Orthosis Options	Goals of Orthosis	Keys to Success
Equinus	HAFO Rigid PLS SAFO	• Provide swing phase clearance • Allow ankle DF as available	• Appropriate evaluation of ankle DF ROM with midfoot position considered • Strong soft tissue support to the midfoot within the AFO
Jump	Rigid PLS SAFO	• Provide swing phase clearance • Accommodate existing plantar flexion contracture • Minimize/eliminate compensatory dorsiflexion at the midfoot • Reestablish function of the PF-KE couple	• Appropriate evaluation of ankle DF ROM with midfoot position considered • Strong soft tissue support to the midfoot within the AFO • Proper alignment of the AFO within the footwear • Adequate stiffness to increase knee extension
Apparent equinus	SAFO FR-AFO	• Provide swing phase clearance • May reestablish heel-first initial contact • Restrict unwanted/excessive tibial progression • Reestablish function of the PF-KE couple	• Appropriate consideration of severity of spasticity • Proper alignment of the AFO within the footwear • Complementary interventions • Adequate stiffness to increase knee extension
Crouch	FR-AFO	• Minimize demand on the quadriceps through reestablishment of the PF-KE • Prevent further progression of lever arm dysfunction	• Appropriate evaluation of ankle DF ROM with midfoot position considered • Consideration of orthopedics for transverse plane bony deformity • Strong soft tissue support to the midfoot within the AFO • Proper alignment of the AFO within the footwear • Adequate stiffness to increase knee extension • Complementary interventions

Abbreviation: DF, dorsiflexion.

overcome the presence of spasticity and plantar flexor contractures. Proper AFO alignment, consideration of ankle dorsiflexion ROM, and complementary management are necessary for most children with CP regardless of the materials or componentry used in the orthotic design.

SUMMARY

Appropriate AFO prescription in ambulatory bilateral CP is driven by the integrity of the PF-KE. Successful AFO prescription requires interaction with complementary interventions. The AFO must accommodate the knee-extended, ankle-isolated, dorsiflexion ROM to optimize knee extension and midfoot integrity. AFO-FC modifications are necessary to reestablish normal gait function and alignment in AFOs designed to improve walking in CP (Table 1).

DISCLOSURE

The investigators have nothing to disclose.

SUPPLEMENTARY DATA

Supplementary data related to this article can be found online at https://doi.org/10.1016/j.pmr.2019.09.007.

REFERENCES

1. Gage JR, Schwartz MH, Koop SE, et al. The identification and treatment of gait problems in cerebral palsy. London: Mac Keith Press; 2009.
2. Hsu JD, Michael JW, Fisk JR, editors. AAOS atlas of orthoses and assistive devices. 4th edition. Philadelphia: Moby Elsevier; 2008.
3. Singerman R, HD, Mansour JM. Design changes in ankle-foot orthosis intended to alter stiffness also alter orthosis kinematics. J Prosthet Orthot 1999;11(3): 48–56.
4. Eddison N, Mulholland M, Chockalingam N. Do research papers provide enough information on design and material used in ankle foot orthoses for children with cerebral palsy? A systematic review. J Child Orthop 2017;11(4):263–71.
5. Eddison N, Chockalingam N. The effect of tuning ankle foot orthoses-footwear combination on the gait parameters of children with cerebral palsy. Prosthet Orthot Int 2013;37(2):95–107.
6. Brehm MA, Harlaar J, Schwartz M. Effect of ankle-foot orthoses on walking efficiency and gait in children with cerebral palsy. J Rehabil Med 2008;40(7):529–34.
7. Ridgewell E, Dobson F, Bach T, et al. A systematic review to determine best practice reporting guidelines for AFO interventions in studies involving children with cerebral palsy. Prosthet Orthot Int 2010;34(2):129–45.
8. Lintanf M, Bourseul JS, Houx L, et al. Effect of ankle-foot orthoses on gait, balance and gross motor function in children with cerebral palsy: a systematic review and meta-analysis. Clin Rehabil 2018;32(9):1175–88.
9. Davids JR, Rowan F, Davis RB. Indications for orthoses to improve gait in children with cerebral palsy. J Am Acad Orthop Surg 2007;15(3):178–88.
10. Gould N, Moreland M, Alvarez R, et al. Development of the child's arch. Foot Ankle 1989;9(5):241–5.
11. Kadhim M, Miller F. Crouch gait changes after planovalgus foot deformity correction in ambulatory children with cerebral palsy. Gait Posture 2014;39(2):793–8.
12. Rodda JM, Graham HK, Carson L, et al. Sagittal gait patterns in spastic diplegia. J Bone Joint Surg Br 2004;86(2):251–8.
13. Bauer J, Patrick Do K, Feng J, et al. Knee recurvatum in children with spastic diplegic cerebral palsy. J Pediatr Orthop 2017. https://doi.org/10.1097/BPO.0000000000000985.
14. Klotz MC, Wolf SI, Heitzmann D, et al. The association of equinus and primary genu recurvatum gait in cerebral palsy. Res Dev Disabil 2014;35(6):1357–63.
15. Bohm H, Matthias H, Braatz F, et al. Effect of floor reaction ankle-foot orthosis on crouch gait in patients with cerebral palsy: What can be expected? Prosthet Orthot Int 2018;42(3):245–53.

16. Rogozinski BM, Davids JR, Davis RB 3rd, et al. The efficacy of the floor-reaction ankle-foot orthosis in children with cerebral palsy. J Bone Joint Surg Am 2009; 91(10):2440–7.

17. Ries AJ, Schwartz MH. Ground reaction and solid ankle-foot orthoses are equivalent for the correction of crouch gait in children with cerebral palsy. Dev Med Child Neurol 2018. https://doi.org/10.1111/dmcn.13999.

18. Schwarze M, Block J, Kunz T, et al. The added value of orthotic management in the context of multi-level surgery in children with cerebral palsy. Gait Posture 2019;68:525–30.

19. Owen E. The importance of being earnest about shank and thigh kinematics especially when using ankle-foot orthoses. Prosthet Orthot Int 2010;34(3): 254–69.

Surgical Tone Reduction in Cerebral Palsy

Sruthi P. Thomas, MD, PhD[a,b], Angela P. Addison, BS[b], Daniel J. Curry, MD[b,*]

KEYWORDS

- Spasticity • Dystonia • Intrathecal baclofen • Deep brain stimulation

KEY POINTS

- Selective dorsal rhizotomy is the optimal surgical tone reducing technique in spastic diplegia with evidence of periventricular leukomalacia on brain MRI.
- Intrathecal baclofen is useful in treating hypertonia for reasons of pain and deformity stabilization/prevention.
- Intrathecal baclofen improves ease of care, either with high cervical catheters for dystonia or lower thoracic catheters for spasticity.
- Deep brain stimulation is reserved in cerebral palsy for mostly dystonic patients where functional improvement of the upper extremities is the goal.

INTRODUCTION

Spasticity can cause muscle stiffness, pain, and discomfort, as well as decreased function. The muscles of individuals with cerebral palsy (CP) are smaller, weaker, and have distinct histologic architecture. Additionally, spasticity leads to shorter muscles, contracture formation, torsion of long bones, and joint degeneration. Children often require multilevel orthopedic surgical intervention, often as single event multilevel surgeries, including soft tissue release, femoral osteotomies, and hip reconstruction.[1] Spasticity is most often problematic in terms of limiting volitional movement and placing the child at risk for deformity with growth over time. It is important, however, to address other characteristics of the child's movement patterns to ascertain if there is significant underlying weakness that may be unmasked if spasticity were dramatically decreased or eliminated. Spasticity also can dampen other forms of hypertonia, particularly dystonia. Most of the time, spasticity reduction is a goal of treatment, but there are instances when spasticity is desirable for functional purposes.

[a] Department of Physical Medicine and Rehabilitation, Baylor College of Medicine, 6701 Fannin Street, Suite 1280, Houston, TX 77030, USA; [b] Department of Neurosurgery, Section of Pediatric Neurosurgery, Baylor College of Medicine, 6701 Fannin Street, Suite 1230, Houston, TX 77030, USA
* Corresponding author.
E-mail address: djcurry@bcm.edu
Twitter: @ThomasMDPhD (S.P.T.)

Phys Med Rehabil Clin N Am 31 (2020) 91–105
https://doi.org/10.1016/j.pmr.2019.09.008
1047-9651/20/© 2019 Elsevier Inc. All rights reserved.

INTRATHECAL BACLOFEN
Overview and Pathophysiology of Intervention

Intrathecal baclofen (ITB) works by activating metabotropic gamma amino butyric acid (GABA) receptors in the brain and spinal cord, which in turn activate G-protein–coupled potassium channels. This allows for the inhibition of the reflex arc within the spinal cord that controls spasticity.[2–4] Intrathecal administration avoids systemic administration that is generally more sedating and requires higher doses of medication.[5] Within the United States, the SynchroMed II Drug Infusion System from Medtronic (Minneapolis, MN) is the predominantly used pump and comes with either a 20-mL or 40-mL reservoir.[6] An ITB reservoir and pump is inserted in the anterior abdominal cavity while an attached catheter is tunneled subcutaneously and then inserted into the intrathecal space with fluoroscopic guidance. The catheter is classically inserted at T8 or T10, but can also be inserted into higher thoracic and cervical regions.[7] One of the benefits of ITB is that it can be infused continuously or with the addition of boluses at particular times of the day, allowing for customization of baclofen dosing for ideal tone management. The initial starting dose is recommended to be twice the effective bolus dose used in the trial delivered over 24 hours (discussed further elsewhere in this article).

Historical Review

ITB was originally used in the spinal cord injury population for spasticity management in 1984.[8] Its use was later expanded to children with spasticity and dystonia secondary to CP with the goal of improving comfort and facilitating gross motor function and personal care.[9]

Ideal Patient Selection

Patient selection is best done in an interdisciplinary clinic setting with specialists from multiple fields, including physiatry, neurosurgery, orthopedics, and neurology. Similar to indications for other antispasticity interventions, the indications for ITB include spasms, pain, progressive deformity, limited ability to transfer, poor sleep, facilitation of personal care, and inefficient gait patterns.[7,10] Although ITB works very effectively to break spasticity, it has also been shown to have significant effects on decreasing dystonia.[10] ITB can be used in a wide range of patients regardless of functionality, from independent to total dependence for activities of daily living. Many consider ITB as being reserved for use in lower functioning individuals with CP, specifically Gross Motor Function Classification System GMFCS IV to V; however, there is utility in its use in the higher functioning, ambulatory population. A retrospective study of ambulatory children with CP who received ITB showed a significant improvement in muscle tone and knee flexion at initial contact in the gait cycle.[11] Further, ITB is typically reserved for diplegic and quadriplegic children as opposed to hemiplegic and triplegic children, because the ITB is thought to cause hypotonia on the unaffected limbs that could affect function. Spasticity management centers are starting to find benefits to ITB in the hemiplegic and triplegic population, as demonstrated by Lai and colleagues[12] in 2008. They reported a case of ITB being applied to a child with spastic hemiplegic CP who had not responded to focal chemical denervation and serial casting, resulting in ankle contracture formation. With the use of ITB, they were able to gain control of the spasticity and prevent recurrence of the contracture after orthopedic correction of the original deformity.

If a patient is deemed an appropriate candidate, then it is recommended that they undergo a trial with a 1-time dose of ITB. In the best case scenario, a patient would be weaned off all other oral antispasticity medications before the trial to avoid any confounders. The initial dose of ITB is 50 μg. If there is no response, the trial can be repeated with 75 and 100 μg. If there is no response after 75 or 100 μg, patients are generally deemed poor candidates for ITB placement. In some cases, clinicians choose to leave a catheter in place so the effects of continuous infusion can be better assessed. This strategy is particularly useful in patients with significant dystonia that can wax and wane. Patients are serially examined after receiving an ITB dose by clinicians, often physiatrists and/or physical therapists, at regular intervals. If a patient's Modified Ashworth Score improves by 2 points, the trial is generally deemed a success.[13] Other considerations for deeming a trial a success include fluidity of movement, decreased muscle spasms, improved range of motion, improved positioning, and increased speed of ambulation.[14]

Complications and Considerations

One of the major benefits of ITB is the ability to titrate the medication to the desired effect.[2] This process can allow for optimal spasticity and dystonia management while preserving head and trunk control. Additionally, the pump can be set to allow for dosing variability and boluses to fine tune needs throughout the day at specific times. A recent systematic review on the effects of ITB found significant improvements in spasticity based on the Modified Ashworth Scale and the Ashworth scale, as well as in dystonia based on the Barry-Albright Dystonia Scale.[15–18] A moderate effect size was found for improvement in gait quality, based on the Gilette Gait Index, and arm/hand function quality, based on the Melbourne Assessment of Unilateral Upper Limb Function.[18–20] Although there are not many studies looking at participation outcomes in this population, there are several smaller studies looking at caregiver burden showing less burden with ITB.[21,22] A small case series showed that children with ITB for spasticity management showed much improved growth in both height and weight despite there being no changes in caloric intake. The researchers theorized that the calories that were going toward involuntary muscle contraction were made available for growth by breaking the spasticity.[23] A study of 100 patients with epilepsy and CP showed a decrease in seizure frequency with ITB.[24]

Although not common, there are some complications from ITB pumps that need to be taken into consideration when implanting. Owing to the relatively rare programming and mechanical pump errors, withdrawal and overdose can both occur and, in some cases, can be fatal if not managed appropriately.[25] Withdrawal is often characterized by hallucination, behavioral changes, hypertension, hyperthermia, and pruritis. While troubleshooting, patients can be managed with GABA-A agonists such as propofol or benzodiazepines. In contrast, baclofen overdose presents with respiratory depression, reduced consciousness, fixed pupils, and hypotension. Unfortunately, there is no pharmacologic intervention to block the effects of baclofen. When overdose is suspected, the pump is turned to minimal settings, giving the patient time to metabolize the baclofen. In the meantime, supportive care is provided, including intubation when necessary.[2] There is also a risk of urinary retention, constipation, hypotonia, rostral progression of weakness and hypothermia directly from the baclofen itself, independent of a pump malfunction.[7]

As with any implanted hardware, there is always a risk of infection and the rates of ITB pump infection are reported to be anywhere from 1% to 9% in the literature.[26–28] Children with spasticity often have significant secondary neuromuscular scoliosis. It is highly debated in the literature whether or not ITB affects the progression of spinal curves, with some saying there is no effect and some saying ITB exacerbates the progression of curves.[29–33] The cost of ITB treatment can be prohibitive, because the surgical costs plus regular reservoir refills are costly.[34] Additionally, ITB pumps require regular physician visits, which can get expensive and require travel and compliance. Although rare, there are also reports of catheter kinks or ruptures, pump migration, pump pocket seroma, pump stalling, and cerebrospinal fluid leaks.[15,20,35–37]

SELECTIVE DORSAL RHIZOTOMY
Overview and Pathophysiology of Intervention

Selective dorsal rhizotomy (SDR) is a neurosurgical procedure for permanent spasticity management. A neurosurgeon identifies the afferent sensory L1 to S2 nerve roots, divides them into rootlets, and cuts the rootlets contributing to aberrant reflex arcs based on neurophysiologic monitoring. Ideally, the neurosurgeon looks for rootlets where a 50-Hz tetanic stimulation at threshold amplitude leads to activation of distant muscle groups or bilateral muscle groups. By eliminating the abnormal reflex arcs in the lumbosacral sensory roots, the neurosurgeon is able to eliminate spasticity without directly affecting the motor nerves. Of note, the pudendal nerve is often monitored and the S2 nerve root is minimally divided to decrease the risk of incontinence and to prevent excessive weakness of the ankle plantarflexors and hip extensors that could lead to a crouch gait.[38]

Historical Review

Foerster[39] performed the first dorsal rhizotomy for spasticity management in 1908.[1] However, he initially completely disconnected the dorsal roots, leading to great improvements in spasticity with the complications of significant muscle weakness as well as loss of sensation and proprioception.[39] Given these complications, the procedure was not used much until the 1960s, when the procedure was modified to only cut a fraction of the dorsal rootlets, thus preserving sensation and proprioception.[40] The addition of intraoperative monitoring was added in 1978 by Fasano and then promoted widely by Peacock and Arens in the 1980s.[40] The classic version of the surgery uses a large L1 to L5 laminectomy or laminoplasty, allowing for full exposure of the nerve roots and more accurate localization of individual nerve roots to specific spinal levels. However, some neurosurgeons have converted to a single-level laminectomy approach to protect children from the long-term effects of extensive spinal surgery while decreasing operative and recovery time.[41–49] Although both approaches are used regularly and the efficacy of both interventions in decreasing spasticity has been proven, there has only been 1 small retrospective case series that compared the 2 surgical variations head to head. This study showed that there was no significant difference in postoperative pain, use of opioids in the postoperative period, or time to mobilization between the 2 techniques. However, the length of hospital stay was 1.8 days shorter when single-level laminectomy was used. Of note, this study did not look at the incidence or progression of scoliosis in these patients.[50] The specificity of individual root stimulation at the level of the conus has not been tested, which is of importance as proximal branches from nerve roots contribute to distal nerve architecture. There may be significant differences in the electrical and physical response to stimulation of the nerve root exiting at the level of the foramen versus at the conus. Further, it is known that anatomic variations exist with a higher than expected incidence.

Ideal Patient Selection

A thorough history and physical examination is essential to the selection process for SDR. The classic patient selected for SDR has spastic diplegic CP (both lower), is ambulatory, and is prepubertal with antigravity strength in the lower extremities. Children under the age of 4 are often not considered for SDR because they are still developing their motor patterns, making it difficult to project their trajectory. In some cases, maturation of motor patterns allows for overcoming abnormal tone such as spasticity and dystonia. Furthermore, a key component to success after SDR is an aggressive physical therapy program to retrain motor patterns, with which most children under 4 years of age would struggle. In contrast, as a child with CP ages, weakness and fixed lower limb deformity become a larger problem.[1,40,42] In some cases, patients may need to be considered for single-event multilevel orthopedic surgery before consideration for SDR for maximum benefit.[51] Children with hemiplegic CP are often skipped over for SDR because it is thought of as a bilateral procedure. Recently, neurosurgeons have been performing hemi-SDR for this population with great success.[52,53] One of the key contraindications to SDR is the coexistence of dystonia or ataxia, because both of these conditions could be exacerbated or unmasked after SDR. Besides physical examination, it is important to get a preoperative MRI of the brain to confirm that there is no injury to the basal ganglia, thalami, brainstem, or cerebellum that could contribute to uncovering dystonia or ataxia after SDR.[38] Generally, patients with severe scoliosis are avoided owing to increased complexity of the surgical approach and a potential risk of worsening scoliosis after SDR. Additionally, patients with significant uncorrected hip subluxation are also excluded owing to the limitations in ambulatory rehabilitation.

Nonambulatory patients are not classically thought of as ideal candidates for SDR. In fact, there are some data that show that SDR leads to minimal gains in functional skills, mobility, and on the Pediatric Evaluation of Disability Inventory in nonambulatory patients.[54] Another study showed that outcomes were poorer in the spastic quadriplegic population compared with the spastic diplegic population.[55] A caveat to these findings is that goals in nonambulatory patients are typically not related to improving mobility, but rather to improving comfort and ease of care as well as preventing progressive deformity. Owing to this intervention requiring 1 surgery and 1 recovery period without risk for malfunction of an implanted device such as with ITB or the need for ongoing maintenance, many families opt for this route to provide permanent tone reduction. Plus, SDR has been shown to be cheaper and less intrusive than ITB while being effective at reducing spasticity and nursing cares.[56] Not only has an improvement been seen in spasticity in the upper and lower extremities, it has been shown to potentially improve bladder dysfunction.[56,57] In cases where there is a concern about dystonia and spasticity being present, a combined motor and sensory rhizotomy can be performed. Because dystonia triggers true muscle contracture, the additional partial disconnection of motor roots decreases dystonia. The drawback is that it weakens the muscle as well, but this is less of a concern in the GMFCS IV and V population that is nonambulatory.[58]

Complications and Considerations

A central key to successful outcomes after SDR is an intensive rehabilitation program, either in the outpatient or inpatient setting.[59] After spasticity has been decreased, muscle weakness is often unmasked and an intensive rehabilitation program is needed for strengthening and gait training.[38]

Ambulatory patients with CP who have undergone SDR have shown improved mobility, endurance, and balance. Together, this leads to decreased falls and improved independence with activities of daily living.[45,60] Individuals who underwent SDR as children showed less functional decline with age, but did not show any differences in pain or fatigue.[61] Furthermore, ambulatory children with CP show significant improvement in functional skills, mobility, and caregiver domains on the Pediatric Evaluation of Disability Inventory after SDR.[54,62] Research is mixed on whether or not SDR prevents future orthopedic interventions.[49,63,64] There are multiple randomized clinical trials that show that SDR plus physical therapy is superior to physical therapy alone.[65–67] A nonrandomized, age and GMFCS matched patient series showed significantly better improvement in Ashworth scores, lower extremity passive range of motion, and Gross Motor Function Measure with SDR compared with ITB.[68] There are some recent long-term studies of the effects of SDR showing continued improvements in range of motion, Gross Motor Function Measure, and multiple domains of the Pediatric Evaluation of Disability Inventory, including self-care and mobility, which showed persistent improvements into early adulthood.[54,62,63]

DEEP BRAIN STIMULATION
Historical Review

Globus pallidus internus deep brain stimulation (DBS) was first performed in a child with generalized dystonia by Coubes and coworkers in 1996.[69] Historically, DBS has been used minimally in the treatment of pediatric movement disorders in general, and CP in particular, for a number of reasons. The most significant reason DBS is not commonly used is that the majority of patients with dystonic CP exhibit a wide spectrum of mixed dystonic and spastic movement characteristics, rather than dystonia alone. DBS specifically targets only dystonia and does not improve spasticity. Dystonia management—surgical or medical—is hampered by a lack of clarity in its diagnosis and classification from other pediatric movement disorders.[70] Outcome measures, such as the Burke-Fahn-Marsden Dystonia Rating Scale (BFMDRS), which was designed for adult generalized dystonia, are difficult to apply meaningfully to dystonic CP and are not validated for children. The effect of DBS on the developing nervous system is not fully known (although experience has shown its relative tolerability) and maintenance of the extension cabling and pulse generating implants have also been difficult to maintain in a axially growing child.[71] DBS has been used more effectively in genetic dystonias such as DYT-1, and somewhat less so in other genetic, degenerative forms of dystonia such as PKAN, Lesch-Nyhan syndrome, glutaric aciduria, and other less globally injured acquired syndromes such as kernicterus. These drawbacks, however, are balanced by the demonstrably poor effect of nonsurgical treatments of childhood dystonia, as elucidated by a published care pathway sponsored by the American Association of Cerebral Palsy and Developmental Medicine showing the possible effectiveness of DBS and ITB in dystonic CP.[72]

There are a number of studies that have investigated the use of DBS in dystonic CP.[73–75] Marks and colleagues[73] showed that DBS in dystonic CP can reduce the BMFDRS motor measure by 37%, but interestingly found that the same treatment only improved the BFMDRS by 8% in the skeletally mature cohort 16 years of age or older. The authors speculated that this may have been due to the BFMDRS decreases being obscured by skeletal contractures. This finding was similar to a small series published by Keen and colleagues,[76] which showed a 30% decrease in the BMFDRS in patients younger than 18 year old. The magnitude of BFMDRS decrease in dystonic CP with DBS was even less in 2 meta-analyses, one of DBS in dystonic CP and another of DBS in general pediatric dystonia, of which dystonic CP was a cohort. Both studies found a mean BFMDRS—movement reduction with DBS of 11%.[77,78] These authors and others point to the insensitivity of the BFMDRS—movement as an outcome measure, and discuss the Canadian Occupational Performance Measure as a possible alternative.[77–79]

Pathophysiology of Intervention

DBS has been used to effectively treat tremors or dystonias in movement disorders such as essential tremor or Parkinson's disease, but its application in pediatrics patients has traditionally been limited. DBS performed by stereotactically implanting electrodes within motor pathway structures beneath the cortex, such as the globus pallidus internus, the subthalamic nucleus, or the ventral intermediate nucleus of the thalamus, and delivering a current controlled by programmable amplitude, frequency, and pulse width.[80] Although the mechanism by which DBS affects the brain is not well-understood in general, or in dystonia in particular, there is some evidence to suggest that it disrupts both normal and abnormal firing patterns of neurons.[81–83] Other compelling evidence suggests that DBS imparts its effect by stimulating the efferent projections from the target nucleus.[84]

Briefly, the basal ganglia circuit (**Fig. 1**) is defined by circuitry from the cortex, projecting to the putamen, and then projecting via direct and indirect pathway from the putamen to the globus pallidus internus and globus pallidus externus, respectively, and from there projecting to the thalamus, and back to the cortex, with collateral involvement of the brainstem and spinal cord.[83] Most cases of CP involve injury to white matter, cerebral cortex, basal ganglia, and/or cerebellum of various degrees.[85] CP-associated movement disorders disrupt motor circuits, either by the cortical-striatal-thalamic-cortical, cortical-cerebellar-cortical, descending motor circuits to the brainstem, or retention of infant reflexes.[85] These areas are more susceptible to

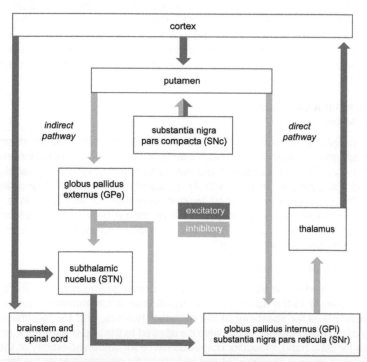

Fig. 1. Schematic of the basal ganglia motor circuit. The motor circuit is defined by the indirect and direct pathways throughout the basal ganglia, and all converge on the globus pallidus internus before final output to the cortex and the brainstem/spinal cord. (*Adapted from* Miocinovic S, Somayajula S, Chitnis S, et al. History, applications, and mechanisms of deep brain stimulation. JAMA Neurol. 2013;70(2):166; with permission.)

injury, depending on the stage of development at the time of the injury; for example, injury to the white matter around the lateral ventricles, termed periventricular leukomalacia, often occurs in preterm birth and imparts motoric spasticity. However, in term infants suffering a hypoxic–ischemic injury, the cerebral cortex, basal ganglia, and the thalamus of the brain are injured, imparting dystonia in addition to spasticity.[85]

Ideal Patient Selection

The ideal dystonic CP patient for DBS remains undefined, but there are some aspects revealed in the meta-analyses that may predict better or worse outcome. The more severely dystonic patients, as revealed by high BFMDRS-M scores, are more likely to have a meager decrease in BFMDRS.[86] The magnitude of the injury, or the multiplicity of structures injured, can also present a challenge.[78] Last, the age of the patient is important, as the intervention must occur prior to contracture formation to maximize the usefulness of the tone reduction.[86] Globus pallidus internus is the most used target, likely owing to its role as the common output of the basal ganglia. If it is injured, the subthalamic nucleus can serve as a target for DBS dystonia control.[87] Others have implanted both targets to maximize the basal ganglia modulation for therapy.[88]

Complications and Considerations

Complications for DBS include the surgical risks such as bleeding, stroke, and component infection, but also include implant erosion, lead or cable fracture, hardware malfunction, bowstringing, and electrode displacement from the target as the patient grows. Koy and colleagues[89] studied the largest cohort of pediatric DBS to date, which showed a remarkably low intracerebral hemorrhage rate of 0.5% per electrode compared with 2.9% per electrode in adults. The infection rate, however, was higher at 12.5% compared with 10% in adults. There was a slight increase in adverse events in the age range of 7- to 9-year-old patients, and after 6 months or more from the operation.

SELECTIVE PERIPHERAL NEUROTOMY
Historical Review

Selective peripheral neurotomy (SPN) is a neurosurgical procedure designed to decrease spasticity surgically and permanently in the muscle groups innervated by the target nerve. The technique was pioneered by Marc Sindou and associates[90] in France and first published in 1985 with 47 cases of tibial nerve SPN for spasticity of the foot. The procedure is designed to decrease harmful spasticity in a regional manner when botulinum toxin injections can no longer be effective. Outcomes can be assessed by measuring the reduction in the Modified Ashworth Score and the passive range of motion of the segment.[91]

Pathophysiology of Intervention

SPN can be applied to the tibial nerve for ankle plantarflexor spasticity, the obturator nerve for spasticity in the adductors, the sciatic nerve for hamstring spasticity, the anterior tibial nerve for spasticity of the extensor hallucis, and the femoral nerve for spasticity of the quadriceps.[92] It can also be applied to the upper extremity, at the median nerve for claw hand, musculocutaneous nerve for flexion spasticity at the elbow, and for relief of internal shoulder rotator spasticity by neurotomies of the lateral pectoral and the lower scapular nerves.[90] The principle is to section 50% to 80% of the nerve branches to a targeted muscle group to be effective but to avoid inducing complete paralysis. Electromyography of the targeted muscles show motor endplates after sectioning and months after the surgery the motor units can be 5 times their original size to compensate for the loss of the motor pool.[93] It can also be combined with tenotomies when muscle tendons are revealed in the exposed surgical field, as is the case in obturator neurotomies.

Ideal Patient Selection

The ideal patient for SPN is suffering from focal spasticity that is medically refractory and resistant to either botulinum toxin injections or phenol injections. It can also be used when 1 segment is disproportionally spastic in patients who are poor candidates for multisegment, spasticity-reducing surgery such as SDR or ITB. It can also serve as a good option when severe tone persists in a specific muscle group, such as hip adductors, after a neurosurgical tone reducing intervention.

Complications and Considerations

SPN has the usual surgical risk of any surgery such as postoperative bleeding or infection. The incisions can frequently be across joint fossa, so wound breakdown complications are possible. Care must be taken to use proper microsurgical technique and electrostimulation to fully dissect the motor branches from the nerve trunks to avoid cutting sensory fibers that could result in deafferentation pain syndromes.[94]

SUMMARY

The management of pathologically increased tone in CP requires complex decision-making that first and foremost focuses on the achievement of the patient's and family's goals of care. Each patient's care plan needs to be tailored to that individual and not addressed dogmatically. Special care needs to be taken to assess a patient's functional hypertonia, the appreciation of which may require a more graduated or adjustable tone reduction strategy. Nonetheless, spasticity and dystonia have both immediate and long-term deleterious effects that need to be addressed early in life to avoid additional surgical interventions, making an aggressive approach warranted. Planning of surgical tone management needs to take into account the care goals, developmental potential, family compliance, continual access to care, and financial resources. The strategy is best planned and performed in a multidisciplinary team composed of physiatrists, neurosurgeons, neurologists, orthopedic surgeons, physical therapists, occupational therapists, and speech therapists, in coordination with the family's primary care physician. Outcomes should be measured objectively through rating scale improvement, but subjective improvements can be just as significant to the patient and family, and therefore deserve continued focus.

Most centers that manage spasticity in patients with CP choose to exhaust nonsurgical options for tone management before considering neurosurgical intervention. Nonsurgical options include oral medications and focal injections with toxins and alcohols. There are some etiologies of hypertonicity, such as severe anoxic brain injury and hypoxic–ischemic encephalopathy, for which surgical tone reduction is considered earlier owing to severe hypertonicity leading to significant patient discomfort, status dystonicus, and also rapidly evolving soft tissue contractures. It is optimal to have all surgical options available for the control of hypertonia, including SDR, ITB, DBS, and SPN. SDR is optimal of ambulatory spastic diplegia patients who exhibit periventricular leukomalacia on their brain MRI and can strengthen in inpatient rehabilitation. ITB has been used in the spasticity management of spastic diplegic patients not fitting the criteria for SDR or in quadriplegic CP, and when the goals are comfort, deformity stabilization, and ease of care. ITB with a high cervical catheter has been used for dystonia management where functional improvement is not expected. DBS is reserved for dystonic CP and disproportionally dystonic mixed tone CP patients where improved upper extremity function is a reasonable goal. Frequently, more than 1 surgical approach is used on the same patient in a staged manner. For instance, severe dystonic CP frequently can undergo ITB for the spastic component and DBS for the dystonic component. SPN is used for segmental spasticity where systemic treatments are either not needed or unnecessarily onus in their commitment.

DISCLOSURE

The authors have nothing to disclose.

REFERENCES

1. Aquilina K, Graham D, Wimalasundera N. Selective dorsal rhizotomy: the re-emergence of an old technique. Arch Dis Child 2015;100:798–802.
2. Roberts A. Surgical management of spasticity. J Child Orthop 2013;7:389–94.
3. Davidoff RA, Hackman JC. GABA: presynaptic actions. In: Rogawski M, editor. Neurotransmitter actions in the vertebrate nervous system. New York: Plenum Press; 1985. p. 3–32.
4. Zieglgansberger W, Howe JR, Sutor B. The neuropharmacology of baclofen. In: Muller H, Zierski J, Penn RD, editors. Local-spinal therapy of spasticity. Berlin: Springer; 1988. p. 37–49.
5. McKinlay I, Hyde E, Gordon N. Baclofen: a team approach to drug evaluation of spasticity in childhood. Scott Med J 1980;25:S26–8.
6. Medtronic. SynchroMed & IsoMed implantable infusion systems. Minneapolis (MN): Author; 2017.
7. Ivanhoe CB, Tilton AH, Francisco GE. Intrathecal baclofen therapy for spastic hypertonia. Phys Med Rehabil Clin N Am 2001;12(4):923–38.
8. Penn R, Kroin J. Continuous intrathecal baclofen for severe spasticity. Lancet 1985;326:125–7.
9. Butler C, Campbell S. Evidence of the effects of intrathecal baclofen for spastic and dystonic cerebral palsy. Dev Med Child Neurol 2000;42:634–45.
10. Albright AL. Intrathecal baclofen in cerebral palsy movement disorders. J Child Neurol 1996;11(S1):S29–35.
11. Pruszczynski B, Sees J, Hulbert R, et al. The effect of continuous intrathecal baclofen therapy on ambulatory children with cerebral palsy. J Pediatr Orthop B 2018;27(3):214–20.
12. Lai LP, Reeves S, Smith BP, et al. Use of intrathecal baclofen in a pediatric cerebral palsy patient with refractory hemiplegia to maintain orthopaedic surgery gains. J Pediatr Rehabil Med 2008;1(3):263–8.
13. Meythaler JM, DeVivo MJ, Hadley M. Prospective study on the use of bolus intrathecal baclofen for spastic hypertonia due to acquired brain injury. Arch Phys Med Rehabil 1996;77:461.
14. Francisco GE. The effect of intrathecal baclofen therapy on walking speed of individuals with post-stroke hemiplegia. Arch Phys Med Rehabil 2000;81:1295.
15. Gray N, Morton RE, Brimlow K, et al. Goals and outcomes for non-ambulant children receiving continuous infusion of intrathecal baclofen. Eur J Paediatr Neurol 2012;16:443–8.
16. Motta F, Stignani C, Antonello CE. The use of intrathecal baclofen pump implants in children and adolescents: safety and complications in 200 consecutive cases. J Neurosurg 2007;107(S1):32–5.

17. Motta F, Stignani C, Antonello CE. Effect of intrathecal baclofen on dystonia in children with cerebral palsy and the use of functional scales. J Pediatr Orthop 2008;28:213–7.

18. Motta F, Antonello CE, Stignani C. Upper limbs function after intrathecal baclofen therapy in children with secondary dystonia. J Pediatr Orthop 2009;29:817–21.

19. Hidalgo ET, Orillac C, Hersh A, et al. Intrathecal baclofen therapy for the treatment of spasticity in Sjogren-Larsson syndrome. J Child Neurol 2017;32:100–3.

20. Brochard S, Remy-Neris O, Filipetti P, et al. Intrathecal baclofen infusion for ambulant children with cerebral palsy. Pediatr Neurol 2009;20:265–70.

21. Hoving MA, van Raak EP, Spincemaille GH, et al. Dutch Study Group on Child Spasticity. Efficacy of intrathecal baclofen therapy in children with intractable spastic cerebral palsy: a randomized controlled trial. Eur J Paediatr Neurol 2009;13:240–6.

22. Vles GF, Soudant DL, Hoving MA, et al. Long-term follow-up on continuous intrathecal baclofen therapy in non-ambulant children with intractable spastic cerebral palsy. Eur J Paediatr Neurol 2013;17(6):639–44.

23. Bottanelli M, Rubini G, Venturelli V, et al. Weight and height gain after intrathecal baclofen pump implantation in children with spastic tetraparesis. Dev Med Child Neurol 2004;46(11):788–9.

24. Buonaguro V, Scelsa B, Curci D, et al. Epilepsy and intrathecal baclofen therapy in children with cerebral palsy. Pediatr Neurol 2005;33(2):110–3.

25. Watve SV, Sivan M, Raza WA, et al. Management of acute overdose or withdrawal state in intrathecal baclofen therapy. Spinal Cord 2012;50(2):107–11.

26. Armstrong RW, Steinbok P, Cochrane DD, et al. Intrathecally administered baclofen for treatment of children with spasticity of cerebral origin. J Neurosurg 1997; 87(3):409–14.

27. Albright AL, Awaad Y, Muhonen M, et al. Performance and complications associated with the synchromed 10-ml infusion pump for intrathecal baclofen administration in children. J Neurosurg 2004;101(S1):64–8.

28. Lam SK, Mayer RR, Vedantam A, et al. Readmission and complications within 30 days after intrathecal baclofen pump placement. Dev Med Child Neurol 2018;60(10):1038–44.

29. Burn SC, Zeller R, Drake JM. Do baclofen pumps influence the development of scoliosis in children? J Neurosurg Pediatr 2010;5(2):195–9.

30. Ginsburg GM, Lauder AJ. Progression of scoliosis in patients with spastic quadriplegia after insertion of an intrathecal baclofen pump. Spine 2007;32(34): 2745–50.

31. Sansone JM, Mann D, Noonan K, et al. Rapid progression of scoliosis following insertion of intrathecal baclofen pump. J Pediatr Orthop 2006;26(1):125–8.

32. Gooch JL, Oberg WA, Grams B, et al. Care provider assessment of intrathecal baclofen in children. Dev Med Child Neurol 2004;46(8):548–52.

33. Shilt JS, Lai LP, Cabrera MN, et al. The impact of intrathecal baclofen on the natural history of scoliosis in cerebral palsy. J Pediatr Orthop 2008;28(6):684–7.

34. Steinbok P, Daneshvar H, Evans D, et al. Cost analysis of continuous intrathecal baclofen versus selective functional posterior rhizotomy in the treatment of spastic quadriplegia associated with cerebral palsy. Pediatr Neurosurg 1995;22(5): 255–64.

35. Walter M, Altermatt S, Furrer C, et al. Intrathecal baclofen therapy in children with severe spasticity: outcome and complications. Dev Neurorehabil 2014;17: 368–74.

36. Murphy NA, Irwin MC, Hoff C. Intrathecal baclofen therapy in children with cerebral palsy: efficacy and complications. Arch Phys Med Rehabil 2002;83:1721–5.
37. Overgard TM, Kjaersgaard-Hansen L, Soe M, et al. Positive experience with intrathecal baclofen treatment in children with severe cerebral palsy. Dan Med J 2015; 62:A4999.
38. Graham D, Aquilina K, Mankad K, et al. Selective dorsal rhizotomy: current state of practice and the role of imaging. Quant Imaging Med Surg 2018;8(2):209–18.
39. Foerster O. The treatment of spastic paralysis by resection of spinal cord roots. Results Surg Orthop 1911;1:174–209.
40. Langerak NG, Lamberts RP, Fieggen AG, et al. Selective dorsal rhizotomy: long-term experience from Cape Town. Childs Nerv Syst 2007;23:1003–6.
41. Park TS, Johnston JM. Surgical techniques of selective dorsal rhizotomy for spastic cerebral palsy. Technical note. Neurosurg Focus 2006;21:e7.
42. Grunt S, Fieggen AG, Vermuelen RJ, et al. Selection criteria for selective dorsal rhizotomy in children with spastic cerebral palsy: a systematic review of the literature. Dev Med Child Neurol 2014;56:302–12.
43. Bolster EA, van Schie PE, Becher JG, et al. Long-term effect of selective dorsal rhizotomy on gross motor function in ambulant children with spastic bilateral cerebral palsy, compared with reference centiles. Dev Med Child Neurol 2013;55: 610–6.
44. Grunt S, Becher JG, Vermuelen RJ. Long-term outcome and adverse effects of selective dorsal rhizotomy in children with cerebral palsy: a systematic review. Dev Med Child Neurol 2011;53:490–8.
45. Langerak NG, Lamberts RP, Fieggen AG, et al. A prospective gait analysis study in patients with diplegic cerebral palsy 20 years after selective dorsal rhizotomy. J Neurosurg Pediatr 2008;1:180–6.
46. Li Z, Zhu J, Liu X. Deformity of lumbar spine after selective dorsal rhizotomy for spastic cerebral palsy. Microsurgery 2008;28:10–2.
47. Steinbok P, Hicdonmez T, Sawatzky B, et al. Spinal deformities after selective dorsal rhizotomy for spastic cerebral palsy. J Neurosurg 2005;102:363–73.
48. Johnson MB, Goldstein L, Thomas SS, et al. Spinal deformity after selective dorsal rhizotomy in ambulatory patients with cerebral palsy. J Pediatr Orthop 2004; 24:529–36.
49. Park TS, Edwards C, Liu JL, et al. Beneficial effects of childhood selective dorsal rhizotomy in adulthood. Cureus 2017;9:e1077.
50. Ou C, Kent S, Miller S, et al. Selective dorsal rhizotomy in children: comparison of outcomes after single-level versus multi-level laminectomy technique. Can J Neurosci Nurs 2010;32(3):17–24.
51. MacWilliams BA, Johnson BA, Shuckra AL, et al. Functional decline in children undergoing selective dorsal rhizotomy after age 10. Dev Med Child Neurol 2011;53:717–23.
52. Zhan Q, Tang L, Wang Y, et al. Feasibility and effectiveness of a newly modified protocol-guided selective dorsal rhizotomy via single-level approach to treat spastic hemiplegia in pediatric cases with cerebral palsy. Childs Nerv Syst 2019. [Epub ahead of print].
53. Fukuhara T, Kamata I. Selective posterior rhizotomy for painful spasticity in the lower limbs of hemiplegic patients after stroke: report of two cases. Neurosurgery 2004;54(5):1268–74.
54. Josenby AL, Wagner P, Jarnlo GB, et al. Functional performance in self-care and mobility after selective dorsal rhizotomy: a 10-year practice-based follow-up study. Dev Med Child Neurol 2015;57:286–93.

55. Kim HS, Steinbok P, Wickenheiser D. Predictors of poor outcome after selective dorsal rhizotomy in treatment of spastic cerebral palsy. Childs Nerv Syst 2006; 22:60–6.

56. Ingale H, Ughratdar I, Muquit S, et al. Selective dorsal rhizotomy as an alternative to intrathecal baclofen pump replacement in GMFCS grades 4 and 5 children. Childs Nerv Syst 2016;32:321–5.

57. D'Aquino D, Moussa AA, Ammar A, et al. Selective dorsal rhizotomy for the treatment of severe spastic cerebral palsy: efficacy and therapeutic durability in GMFCS grade IV and V children. Acta Neurochir 2018;160:811–21.

58. Ghany WAA, Nada M, Mahran MA, et al. Combined anterior and posterior lumbar rhizotomy for treatment of mixed dystonia and spasticity in children with cerebral palsy. Neurosurgery 2016;79(3):336–43.

59. Graham D, Aquilina K, Cawker S, et al. Single-level selective dorsal rhizotomy for spastic cerebral palsy. J Spine Surg 2016;2:195–201.

60. Chicoine MR, Park TS, Kaufman BA. Selective dorsal rhizotomy and rates of orthopaedic surgery in children with spastic cerebral palsy. J Neurosurg 1997; 86:34–9.

61. Daunter AK, Kratz AL, Hurvitz EA. Long-term impact of childhood selective dorsal rhizotomy on pain, fatigue, and function: a case-control study. Dev Med Child Neurol 2017;59:1089–95.

62. Nordmark E, Josenby AL, Lagergren J, et al. Long-term outcomes five years after selective dorsal rhizotomy. BMC Pediatr 2008;8:54.

63. Dudley RW, Parolin M, Gagnon B, et al. Long-term functional benefits of selective dorsal rhizotomy for spastic cerebral palsy. J Neurosurg Pediatr 2013;12:142–50.

64. Watt JM, Robertson CM, Grace MG. Early prognosis for ambulation of neonatal intensive care survivors with cerebral palsy. Dev Med Child Neurol 1989;31: 766–73.

65. Wright FV, Sheil EM, Drake JM, et al. Evaluation of selective dorsal rhizotomy for the reduction of spasticity in cerebral palsy: a randomized controlled trial. Dev Med Child Neurol 1998;40(4):239–47.

66. Steinbok P, Reiner AM, Beauchamp R, et al. A randomized clinical trial to compare selective posterior rhizotomy plus physiotherapy with physiotherapy alone in children with spastic diplegic cerebral palsy. Dev Med Child Neurol 1997;39(3): 178–84.

67. McLaughlin JF, Bjornson KF, Astley SJ, et al. Selective dorsal rhizotomy: efficacy and safety in an investigator-masked randomized clinical trial. Dev Med Child Neurol 1998;40(4):220–32.

68. Kan P, Gooch J, Amini A, et al. Surgical treatment of spasticity in children: comparison of selective dorsal rhizotomy and intrathecal baclofen pump implantation. Childs Nerv Syst 2008;24(2):239–43.

69. Coubes P, Echenne B, Roubertie A, et al. Treatment of early-onset generalized dystonia by chronic bilateral stimulation of the internal globus pallius: Apropos a case. Neurochirurgie 1999;45(2):139–44.

70. Eggink H, Kremer D, Brouwer OF, et al. Spasticity, dyskinesia and ataxia in cerebral palsy: are we sure we can differentiate them? Eur J Paediatr Neurol 2017; 21(5):703–6.

71. Marks WA, Honeycutt J, Acosta F, et al. Deep brain stimulation for pediatric movement disorders. Semin Pediatr Neurol 2009;16(2):90–8.

72. Fehlings D, Brown L, Harvey A, et al. Pharmacological and neurosurgical interventions for managing dystonia in cerebral palsy: a systematic review. Dev Med Child Neurol 2018;60(4):356–66.

73. Marks WA, Honeycutt J, Acosta F Jr, et al. Dystonia due to cerebral palsy responds to deep brain stimulation of the globus pallidus internus. Mov Disord 2011;26(9):1748–51.

74. Air EL, Ostrem JL, Sanger TD, et al. Deep brain stimulation in children: experience and technical pearls. J Neurosurg Pediatr 2011;8(6):566–74.

75. Olaya JE, Christian E, Ferman D, et al. Deep brain stimulation in children and young adults with secondary dystonia: the Children's Hospital Los Angeles experience. Neurosurg Focus 2013;35(5):E7.

76. Keen JR, Przekop A, Olaya JE, et al. Deep brain stimulation for the treatment of childhood dystonic cerebral palsy. J Neurosurg Pediatr 2014;14(6):585–93.

77. Koy A, Hellmich M, Pauls KA, et al. Effects of deep brain stimulation in dyskinetic cerebral palsy: a meta-analysis. Mov Disord 2013;28(5):647–54.

78. Elkaim LM, Alotaibi NM, Sigal A, et al, North American Pediatric DBS Collaboration. Deep brain stimulation for pediatric dystonia: a meta-analysis with individual participant data. Dev Med Child Neurol 2019;61(1):49–56.

79. Gimeno H, Tustin K, Lumsden D, et al. Evaluation of functional goal outcomes using the Canadian Occupational Performance Measure (COPM) following Deep Brain Stimulation (DBS) in childhood dystonia. Eur J Paediatr Neurol 2014; 18(3):308–16.

80. Coffey RJ. Deep brain stimulation devices: a brief technical history and review. Artif Organs 2009;33:208–20.

81. Perlmutter JS, Mink JW. Deep brain stimulation. Annu Rev Neurosci 2006;29: 229–57.

82. Gradinaru V, Mogri M, Thompson KR, et al. Optical deconstruction of Parkinsonian neural circuitry. Science 2009;324:354–9.

83. Miocinovic S, Somayajula S, Chitnis S, et al. History, applications, and mechanisms of deep brain stimulation. JAMA Neurol 2013;70:163–71.

84. Anderson ME, Postnupa N, Ruffo M. Effects of high-frequency stimulation in the internal globus pallidus on the activity of thalamic neurons in the awake monkey. J Neurophysiol 2013;89:1150–60.

85. Graham HK, Rosenbaum P, Paneth N, et al. Cerebral palsy. Nat Rev Dis Primers 2016;2:15082.

86. Cif L, Coubes P. Historical developments in children's deep brain stimulation. Eur J Paediatr Neurol 2017;21(1):109–17.

87. Ostrem JL, San Luciano M, Dodenhoff KA, et al. Subthalamic nucleus deep brain stimulation in isolated dystonia: a 3-year follow-up study. Neurology 2017;88(1): 25–35.

88. Sanger TD, Liker M, Arguelles E, et al. Pediatric deep brain stimulation using awake recording and stimulation for target selection in an inpatient neuromodulation monitoring unit. Brain Sci 2018;8(7):E135.

89. Koy A, Bockhorn N, Kühn AA, et al. GEPESTIM consortium. Adverse events associated with deep brain stimulation in patients with childhood-onset dystonia. Brain Stimul 2019;12(5):1111–20.

90. Sindou MP, Simon F, Mertens P, et al. Selective peripheral neurotomy (SPN) for spasticity in childhood. Childs Nerv Syst 2007;23(9):957–70.

91. Sitthinamsuwan B, Chanvanitkulchai K, Phonwijit L, et al. Surgical outcomes of microsurgical selective peripheral neurotomy for intractable limb spasticity. Stereotact Funct Neurosurg 2013;91(4):248–57.

92. Decq P, Filipetti P, Feve A, et al. Selective peripheral neurotomy of the hamstring branches of the sciatic nerve in the treatment of spastic flexion of the knee. Apropos of a series of 11 patients. Neurochirurgie 1996;42(6):275–80.

93. Sindou M, Abdennebi B, Sharkey P. Microsurgical selective procedures in peripheral nerves and the posterior root-spinal cord junction for spasticity. Appl Neurophysiol 1985;48(1–6):97–104.
94. Deltombe T, Detrembleur C, Hanson P, et al. Selective tibial neurotomy in the treatment of spastic equinovarus foot: a 2-year follow-up of three cases. Am J Phys Med Rehabil 2006;85(1):82–8.

The Role of Motion Analysis in Surgical Planning for Gait Abnormalities in Cerebral Palsy

Eric L. Dugan, PhD[a,b,*], Jeffrey S. Shilt, MD[a,b]

KEYWORDS

- Classification • Treatment • Kinematics • SEMLS

KEY POINTS

- Gait deviations in cerebral palsy are complex and difficult to characterize.
- Clinical gait analysis is composed of 2 primary components: data collection and data interpretation.
- Clinical gait analysis facilitates presurgical decision making.

INTRODUCTION

"First, do no harm" is a phrase well known to all who practice medicine.[1] Although the cause is less certain, the intent is well understood. As such, ensuring quality in medicine has been at the forefront of medical practice for centuries. Attention has been focused on creating objective measurement of quality outcomes for the past 2 decades. This focus is highlighted by the Institute of Medicine (renamed in 2015 the National Academy of Medicine) publication of 2 reports: *To Err is Human*[2] and *Crossing the Quality Chasm*.[3] The latter included 6 aims, the first 2 of which are related to the quality domains of safety and effectiveness. Safety is defined as avoiding harm to patients from the care that is intended to help them, and effectiveness as providing services based on scientific knowledge to all who could benefit and refraining from providing services to those not likely to benefit, thereby avoiding underuse and misuse, respectively.

Gait abnormalities in cerebral palsy are complex and difficult to accurately characterize. As such, clinical gait analysis was introduced as an effort to address the deficiencies and shortcomings in the surgical management of cerebral palsy based on observation. Gage[4] introduced the use of gait analysis to better understand the complex array of primary and secondary functional problems often associated with

[a] Department of Orthopedic Surgery, Baylor College of Medicine, 7200 Cambridge, Ste. 10A, Houston, TX 77030, USA; [b] Texas Children's Hospital, 17580 Interstate 45 South, The Woodlands, TX 77384, USA
* Corresponding author. Texas Children's Hospital, 17580 Interstate 45 South, The Woodlands, TX 77384.
E-mail address: eldugan@texaschildrens.org

Phys Med Rehabil Clin N Am 31 (2020) 107–115
https://doi.org/10.1016/j.pmr.2019.09.009
1047-9651/20/© 2019 Elsevier Inc. All rights reserved.

cerebral palsy. The premise was that primary deformities should be treated, whereas secondary compensations should not because they often resolve once the primary abnormality is addressed.[4]

Incorrect treatment can result in harm manifested by loss of function, unnecessary surgery, decreased quality of life, and increased cost. Therefore, treatment interventions directed toward improving gait abnormalities in cerebral palsy should be based on reliable information in order to provide both safe and effective care. Ultimately, the challenges facing the clinical gait analysis community are 2-fold:

1. Collection of accurate and reliable data
2. Development of effective treatment strategies derived (at least in part) from motion analysis data

In Baker's[5] review of clinical gait analysis, he describes the current state of gait analysis as existing on a spectrum from the objective process of data collection to the subjective process of clinical interpretation.

DATA COLLECTION

Some people may be surprised that the history of gait analysis reaches back to Aristotle (384–322 BC), who described the vertical oscillations of the head during gait. Since that time, technologic advances have made motion analysis increasingly objective and clinically relevant. Some key benchmarks in this progression include the development of photographic methods by Muybridge and Stanford in 1878 to more objectively assess two-dimensional kinematics; the first three-dimensional gait analysis by Otto Fischer and Willhelm Brane in the late 1800s; Elftmans' development of the three-dimensional force plate, allowing the study of gait kinetics; Verne Inman's work at the University of Berkeley following World War II; and the work of Jacqueline Perry and Donald Sutherland in the development of the clinical gait analysis in the 1960s. For a complete history of the technical aspects of gait analysis, the authors recommend Richard Baker's[6] review of the topic.

The motion analysis laboratory at Newington Children's Hospital led by Dr James Gage transformed motion analysis into a more readily available tool for clinical use by computerizing the tedious processing of cine film, greatly increasing the speed with which the data could be reviewed. Motion analysis of gait now consists of state-of-the-art three-dimensional motion capture systems, force plates, and electromyography with processing software that integrates kinematics (joint angles), kinetics (ground reaction forces), electromyogram (muscle activity), and pedobarography (foot pressure data) to quantify gait dysfunction. Accurate and reliable collection of data is now achievable and is no longer a significant source of error in clinical gait analysis.[5] In addition, an accreditation body, the Commission for Motion Laboratory Accreditation, has been established to verify that motion analysis laboratories adhere to established standards.

USING MOTION ANALYSIS DATA

It has been shown that instrumented gait analysis does influence treatment plans. Wren and colleagues[7] reported that changes were recommended in the surgical plans for 86% of patients following gait analysis. Furthermore, in 97% of those patients, at least 1 of the recommended changes was implemented. In a study by Lofterød and colleagues,[8] approximately 70% of patients had treatment plans changed following gait analysis. These studies highlight the disparity between treatment plans derived from traditional clinical evaluations and those from gait analyses. This finding is in accordance with Gage's[4] assertion that clinical evaluations alone are not sufficient to understand the complexities of gait disorders associated with cerebral palsy.

However, in order for clinical gait analysis to gain widespread acceptance, it must meet the clinical test criteria described by Brand[9] and later modified by Baker.[5] Specifically, for gait analysis to be used as a clinical test, Baker[5] asserts that it should contribute to the determination of the appropriate intervention (or nonintervention) based on the ability to:

1. Diagnose between disease entities
2. Assess severity, extent, or nature of a disease or injury
3. Monitor progress in the presence or absence of intervention
4. Predict the outcome of intervention or nonintervention

DIAGNOSIS AND CLASSIFICATION OF GAIT PATTERNS

Much of the early work in gait analysis was focused on classifying gait patterns and the degree of impairment, which is consistent with the first 2 components described by Brand[9] and Baker.[5] This work has led to a much better understanding of the functional impairments associated with cerebral palsy and has provided a common vocabulary to describe and classify these impairments.

Approximately 30 years ago, 4 principal types of hemiplegic gait were described based on lower extremity sagittal plane kinematics by Gage[4] and Winters and colleagues.[10] The patterns range from least involvement (type I) to most involvement (type IV), with each subsequent classification building on the former. Type I is characterized by foot drop, increased knee flexion at initial contact, increased hip flexion, and increased lordosis. Type II gait pattern includes all deviations present in type I plus increases in plantarflexion and knee hyperextension. Type III gait pattern includes all deviations in types I and II along with decreased motion. In addition, type IV is a combination of all previous deviations plus decreased hip motion and increased lordosis. At this time, Gage[4] did not present any classification system for diplegic gait patterns because of the complexity of those patterns and impairments.[4,10]

In 2001, Rodda and Graham[11] proposed a classification for both spastic hemiplegia and diplegia as a means of developing a treatment algorithm. The classification system consisted of 4 types of hemiplegic and 4 types of diplegic postural pattern. The term postural patterns was used to described postures typically present in midstance to late stance as opposed to classifications based on joint or segment angle graphs of the entire gait cycle. Similar to the system described by Gage[4] and Winters and colleagues,[10] the hemiplegic patterns were divided into 4 categories: (1) drop foot, (2) true equinus with or without knee hyperextension, (3) true equinus with jump knee, and (4) equinus with jump knee and frontal and transverse plane hip rotation. In addition, diplegic patterns were described as (1) true equinus, (2) jump knee, (3) apparent equinus, and (4) crouch gait.

These early classification systems provided a common vocabulary to describe and classify gait patterns and impairments associated with typical gait patterns observed in patients with cerebral palsy; however, they had some inherent shortcomings. For example, they were (1) based almost entirely on sagittal plane kinematics, (2) based on arbitrary descriptions and therefore not always clinically relevant, and (3) not reliable.[12]

In response to the shortcomings of these early classification schemes, Davids and Bagley[13] proposed a system to classify gait patterns based on stance and swing phase gait deviations. Although this classification scheme used some of the same terminology of the previous systems, it had the advantage of incorporating both transverse plane kinematics and relevant kinetics. Another useful component of this scheme is that it is based on gait deviations and associated impairments rather than strictly describing observed patterns. This property allows the classification system to be applied to both hemiplegic and diplegic patients.

DETERMINATION OF TREATMENT METHODS AND PREDICTING OUTCOMES

The third and fourth components of clinical tests described by Brand[9] and Baker[5] are not as well documented in the gait analysis literature, in large part because of the diversity of treatment approaches for gait-related impairments in cerebral palsy. The lack of common treatment practices complicates the process of developing predicative algorithms for treatment planning; there is less known about the indications and contraindications that allow clinicians to reliably choose interventions that lead to good outcomes while avoiding treatment interventions that lead to poor outcomes.

Much of what is known about treatment interventions and outcomes is derived from the implementation and study of single-event multilevel surgery (SEMLS). as first described by Norlin and Tkaczuk,[14] SEMLS has gained widespread acceptance and is considered by most clinicians as best practice.[15,16] The SEMLS approach involves addressing 2 or more levels of musculoskeletal disorder in 1 operative session. The primary advantage of SEMLS is that the patient only must undergo 1 hospitalization and rehabilitation period. In terms of outcomes, SEMLS has been shown to improve knee and ankle kinematics and improve transverse plane kinematics related to lever-arm dysfunction,[15] and there is evidence that SEMLS leads to changes in gait patterns.[17]

Research on the effectiveness of SEMLS has also led to a better understanding of which patients are likely to benefit most from SEMLS and is laying the foundation for the ability to predict outcomes of surgical interventions. For example, the age at surgery has been shown to be a good predictor of SEMLS outcomes, with patients between the ages of 10 and 12 years having the best outcomes.[18] It has also been shown that patients with the most abnormal gait patterns, as measured by a summary statistic, show the greatest improvement following SEMLS.[19] Edwards and colleagues[20] found that age, Gross Motor Functional Classification System (GMFCS) level, and preoperative gait profile score were the best predictors of improvement following SEMLS. Based on their review, the authors suggest that patients between the ages of 10 and 12 years with GMFCS level II and low gait profile scores are likely to experience the best outcomes following SEMLS.

Although this progress is promising, there are limitations to the current state of SEMLS-related research. First, most of the research conducted on SEMLS outcomes is level 3 or 4 based on the Oxford Centre for Evidence-Based Medicine scale.[15,16] Another weakness of the current literature base is that many of the SEMLS studies do not report their negative outcomes, which compromises the ability to develop contraindications for surgical interventions.[16] This weakness was supported by a recent meta-analysis, in which only 23% of studies adequately reported adverse events.[17]

Although there is ample evidence to support the premise that clinical gait analysis can be used to inform treatment, and predict and track outcomes, the complex nature of SEMLS, including the diversity of the specific components of the SEMLS procedure and the lack of consistency in reporting of rehabilitation protocols, it is still difficult to predict outcomes for individual procedures and thus it is difficult to develop treatment algorithms for specific surgical interventions.[17,21]This difficulty leads to variability in clinical recommendations and has led to some investigators to question the utility or necessity of clinical gait analysis.[22,23]

The question of repeatability both within an institution and between institutions has been addressed using common datasets. Skaggs and colleagues[24] examined the variability in clinical interpretation of clinical gait analysis data across 12 different reviewers at 6 institutions. Each of the orthopedic surgeons reviewed gait studies from 7 different patients and identified the problems that contributed to the patients' gait patterns and also indicated their recommended interventions. The kappa values ranged from 0.11 to 0.64, indicating slight to substantial reliability across the surgical recommendations. Similarly, Wang and colleagues[25] examined the consistency of problem identification and treatment recommendations within an institution. Seven different orthopedic surgeons independently reviewed clinical gait analysis data from 15 patients and were asked to identify gait problems and associated treatment recommendations. The average kappa value for the top 10 recommended treatments was 0.59, which represents moderate agreement.

Although these kappa values may seem low, it is important to view them in context. As both Skaggs and colleagues[24] and Wang and colleagues[25] point out, the values obtained in their studies are consistent with, and often higher than, those of other clinical classification systems.

The topic of how clinical gait analysis is regarded in terms of evidence of its usefulness is addressed very well by Thomason and colleagues[26] who in their commentary about the role of clinical gait analysis in the planning of SEMLS. They make the case that clinical gait analyses provide reliable, valid measures of gait function, but these data do not inherently provide specific surgical recommendations. On the contrary, the choice of surgical intervention is influenced by surgeons' training, institutional biases, and regional biases. Those who question the usefulness of clinical gait analysis are often holding it to a higher standard than other analogous assessments and conflating the difference between the clinical gait analysis data and the recommendations derived from those data.

CLINICAL DECISION MAKING USING MOTION ANALYSIS DATA

To address the variability in clinical decision making, a standard algorithmic approach is needed to facilitate consistency. To this end, several investigators have proposed approaches to the clinical decision-making process. For example, Novacheck and Gage[27] presented 5 management principles for addressing gait disorder in cerebral palsy: (1) spasticity reduction, (2) correction of contractures, (3) simplification of the control system, (4) preservation of power generators, and (5) correction of lever-arm dysfunction. Miller[28] published a decision tree that provided recommended interventions based on level of involvement, gait pattern, physical examination findings, and gait analysis results. Baker[29] developed an impairment-based approach to clinical gait analysis interpretation that focuses on identifying gait deviations and associated impairments. Each of these approaches provides a useful framework for the interpretation of clinical gait analysis data and subsequent clinical decisions. They are not mutually exclusive and often are used in conjunction either explicitly or implicitly.

A diagnostic matrix, as described by Davids and colleagues,[30] is a particularly useful paradigm for the integration of information from multiple sources to guide clinical decision making. Clinical gait analyses include more than just the kinematic, kinetic, electromyographic, and pedobarographic data. These data are typically complemented by a physical examination, radiographs, and two-dimensional video. Each of these components provides a different but complementary piece of information about the patients' ambulatory status and function. The diagnostic matrix as first proposed by Davids and colleagues[30] is based on integrating the different sources of information obtained from an individual's: (1) clinical history, (2) physical examination, (3) diagnostic imaging, (4) examination under anesthesia, and (5) quantitative gait analysis. This matrix was later modified to include individuals' (1) clinical history, (2) physical examination, (3) radiographs, (4) observational gait analysis, and (5) quantitative gait analysis.[31] This system is also compatible with the frameworks described by Novacheck and Gage,[27] Miller,[28] and Baker.[29]

The advantage of using a matrix approach is that it allows the integration of different types of data to drive decision making. The relative confidence of a particular intervention recommendation should be proportionate to the consistency of the data in the matrix. When inconsistencies arise across the data in relation to a specific gait problem, the data type that is considered most valid and reliable should be used to inform the intervention recommendation.[30] It is important to consider all data sources because each source has its own strengths, weaknesses, and limitations. Each of these components provides a different but complementary piece of information about each patient's ambulatory status and function. Interpretation of the data is typically conducted by a team of clinical and technical experts and involves collaborative decision making about recommended treatment interventions. By reviewing all data sources in concert, it is more likely to distinguish between the patients' primary gait impairments and other secondary and tertiary deviations[30,32,33] that should not be addressed surgically. Because the clinical questions vary between patients, the sources best suited to address clinical decisions may vary also. An example of this type of approach applied to selective dorsal rhizotomy cases is provided by van der Krogt and colleagues.[34]

FUTURE DIRECTIONS

The process of integrating data from multiple sources and assessing for patterns is challenging; however, it may be possible to leverage statistical modeling or machine learning to assist with the process of clinical decision making. For example, Schwartz and colleagues[35] used random forest algorithms with large datasets to determine surgical indications and prediction of outcomes for femoral derotation osteotomies and iliopsoas lengthenings.[36] Machine learning algorithms have also been used to classify gait patterns based on a plantarflexion–knee extension couple index,[37] predict GMFCS level,[38] and better describe gait patterns and level of impairment in crouch gait.[39] These uses of large datasets and machine learning approaches and others show promise in aiding in the development of clinical intervention algorithms.

SUMMARY

Gait abnormalities in cerebral palsy are complex and difficult to accurately characterize. Clinical gait analysis shows the prerequisite components of a clinical test to aid in the treatment planning for patients with cerebral palsy. Clinical gait analysis can be used to distinguish between different levels of impairment, can be used to monitor progress and outcomes, and is beginning to show promise for prediction of postsurgical outcomes. Clinical gait analysis can also provide important and relevant information for treatment planning, enhance the likelihood of positive outcomes, and reduce the number of negative outcomes.

DISCLOSURE

The authors have no commercial or financial interests to disclose.

REFERENCES

1. Smith C. Origin and uses of primum non Nocere—Above all, do no harm. J Clin Pharmacol 2005;45(4):371–7. Available at: http://ovidsp.ovid.com/ovidweb.cgi?T=JS&NEWS=n&CSC=Y&PAGE=fulltext&D=ovft&AN=00004700-200504000-00002.
2. Institute of Medicine. To Err Is Human: Building a Safer Health System. Washington, DC: The National Academies Press; 2000. https://doi.org/10.17226/9728.
3. Institute of Medicine. Crossing the Quality Chasm: A New Health System for the 21st Century. Washington, DC: The National Academies Press; 2001. https://doi.org/10.17226/10027.
4. Gage JR. Gait analysis. an essential tool in the treatment of cerebral palsy. Clin Orthop Relat Res 1993;(288):126–34.
5. Baker R. Gait analysis methods in rehabilitation. J Neuroeng Rehabil 2006;3(1):4.
6. Baker R. The history of gait analysis before the advent of modern computers. Gait Posture 2007;26(3):331–42.
7. Wren TAL, Elihu KJ, Mansour S, et al. Differences in implementation of gait analysis recommendations based on affiliation with a gait laboratory. Gait Posture 2012;37(2):206–9.
8. Lofterød B, Terjesen T, Skaaret I, et al. Preoperative gait analysis has a substantial effect on orthopedic decision making in children with cerebral palsy: comparison between clinical evaluation and gait analysis in 60 patients. Acta Orthop 2007;78(1):74–80.
9. Brand RA. Can Biomechanics Contribute to Clinical Orthopaedic Assessments? The Iowa Orthopaedic Journal 1989;9:61–4.
10. Winters TF, Gage JR, Hicks R. Gait patterns in spastic hemiplegia in children and young adults. J Bone Joint Surg Am 1987;69(8):1304.
11. Rodda J, Graham HK. Classification of gait patterns in spastic hemiplegia and spastic diplegia: a basis for a management algorithm. Eur J Neurol 2001;8(s5):98–108.
12. Dobson F, Morris ME, Baker R, et al. Gait classification in children with cerebral palsy: a systematic review. Gait Posture 2006;25(1):140–52.
13. Davids J,R, Bagley A. Identification of common gait disruption patterns in children with cerebral palsy. J Am Acad Orthop Surg 2014;22(12):782–90.
14. Norlin R, Tkaczuk H. One-session surgery for correction of lower extremity deformities in children with cerebral palsy. J Pediatr Orthop 1985;5(2):208–11.
15. Lamberts RP, Burger M, du Toit J, et al. A systematic review of the effects of single-event multilevel surgery on gait parameters in children with spastic cerebral palsy. PLoS One 2016;11(10):e0164686.
16. McGinley JL, Dobson F, Ganeshalingam R, et al. Single-event multilevel surgery for children with cerebral palsy: a systematic review. Dev Med Child Neurol 2012;54(2):117–28.
17. Amirmudin NA, Lavelle G, Theologis T, et al. Multilevel surgery for children with cerebral palsy: a meta-analysis. Pediatrics 2019;143(4):e20183390.
18. Švehlík M, Steinwender G, Lehmann T, et al. Predictors of outcome after single-event multilevel surgery in children with cerebral palsy: a retrospective ten-year follow-up study. Bone Joint J 2016;98-B(2):278–81.
19. Rutz E, Donath S, Tirosh O, et al. Explaining the variability improvements in gait quality as a result of single event multi-level surgery in cerebral palsy. Gait Posture 2013;38(3):455–60.

20. Edwards TA, Theologis T, Wright J. Predictors affecting outcome after single-event multilevel surgery in children with cerebral palsy: a systematic review. Dev Med Child Neurol 2018;60(12):1201–8.

21. Jea A, Dormans J. Single-event multilevel surgery: contender or pretender. Pediatrics 2019;143(4):e20190102.

22. Narayanan U. Management of children with ambulatory cerebral palsy: an evidence-based review. J Pediatr Orthop 2012;32(Suppl 2):S17–181.

23. Noonan K, Halliday S, Browne R, et al. Interobserver variability of gait analysis in patients with cerebral palsy. J Pediatr Orthop 2003;23(3):279–87.

24. Skaggs D, Rethlefsen S, Kay R, et al. Variability in gait analysis interpretation. J Pediatr Orthop 2000;20(6):759–64.

25. Wang KK, Stout JL, Ries AJ, et al. Interobserver reliability in the interpretation of three-dimensional gait analysis in children with gait disorders. Dev Med Child Neurol 2018. https://doi.org/10.1111/dmcn.14051.

26. Thomason P, Rodda J, Sangeux M, et al. Management of children with ambulatory cerebral palsy: an evidence-based review. commentary by hugh williamson gait laboratory staff. J Pediatr Orthop 2012;32(Suppl 2):S18–186.

27. Novacheck T, Gage J. Orthopedic management of spasticity in cerebral palsy. Childs Nerv Syst 2007;23(9):1015–31.

28. Miller F. Cerebral palsy. New York: Springer; 2005.

29. Baker R. Measuring walking : a handbook of clinical gait analysis. London: Mac Keith Press; 2013. Available at: https://ebookcentral.proquest.com/lib/[SITE_ID]/detail.action?docID=1622917.

30. Davids J,R, Ounpuu S, DeLuca PA, et al. Optimization of walking ability of children with cerebral palsy. J Bone Joint Surg 2003;85(11):2224–34.

31. Davids JR. Biomechanically based clinical decision making in pediatric foot and ankle surgery. In: Sabharwal S, editor. Pediatric lower limb deformities: principles and techniques of management. 1st edition. Cham (Switzerland): Springer; 2015. Available at: https://ebookcentral.proquest.com/lib/[SITE_ID]/detail.action?docID=4091073.

32. Sangeux M, Armand S. Kinematic deviations in children with cerebral palsy Orthopedic management of children with cerebral palsy: A comprehensive approach. Nova Science Publishers Inc; 2015. p. 567. Available at: https://archive-ouverte.unige.ch/unige:81177.

33. Schmid S, Schweizer K, Romkes J, et al. Secondary gait deviations in patients with and without neurological involvement: a systematic review. Gait Posture 2012;37(4):480–93.

34. van der Krogt M, van Hutten K, Harlaar J, et al. A systematic clinical reasoning tool to support gait analysis interpretation: an SDR case example. Gait Posture 2017;57:368–9.

35. Schwartz MH, Rozumalski A, Novacheck TF. Femoral derotational osteotomy: surgical indications and outcomes in children with cerebral palsy. Gait Posture 2013; 39(2):778–83.

36. Schwartz MH, Rozumalski A, Truong W, et al. Predicting the outcome of intramuscular psoas lengthening in children with cerebral palsy using preoperative gait data and the random forest algorithm. Gait Posture 2012;37(4):473–9.

37. Sangeux M, Rodda J, Graham HK. Sagittal gait patterns in cerebral palsy: the plantarflexor–knee extension couple index. Gait Posture 2015;41(2):586–91.

38. Schwartz MH, Munger ME. ESMAC BEST PAPER 2017: using machine learning to overcome challenges in GMFCS level assignment. Gait Posture 2018;63:290.
39. Rozumalski A, Schwartz MH. Crouch gait patterns defined using k-means cluster analysis are related to underlying clinical pathology. Gait Posture 2009;30(2): 155–60.

Technological Advancements in Cerebral Palsy Rehabilitation

Fabiola Reyes, MD[a],*, Christian Niedzwecki, DO[a],
Deborah Gaebler-Spira, MD[b]

KEYWORDS

- Rehabilitation robotics • Virtual reality
- Augmentative and alternative communication technology • Mobile applications
- Rehabilitation technology

KEY POINTS

- Robotics in the cerebral palsy rehabilitation arena is a rapidly growing field that can be applied to address impairments in gait, limb movements, self-care, and motivation.
- Rehabilitation principles of neuroplasticity and motivation can be applied through virtual reality, which provides real-time movement feedback and simulates real-life and entertaining environments.
- Technological advances have allowed for more compact and accessible augmentative and alternative communication devices, providing easier means of communication for individuals who may need specialized tools to communicate.
- Resources that help patients with cerebral palsy, their families, and clinicians are available through mobile applications and can provide educational and management tools in many settings.
- Accurate nomenclature and robust protocols and outcome measures can help strengthen studies, which are needed to validate rehabilitation technologies.

INTRODUCTION

In the last decade, technology applications in the field of neurorehabilitation have grown at a rapid pace. This growth is driven by robust engineering research, commercial development of neurorehabilitation products, and through new applications of rapidly expanding technological advances to the field of health care.[1–3] As a result,

Disclosure Statement: D. Gaebler-Spira is a consultant for Rehabtek, a rehabilitation robotics company. The other authors have nothing to disclose.
[a] H. Ben Taub Department of Physical Medicine and Rehabilitation, Baylor College of Medicine, Texas Children's Hospital, 6701 Fannin Street, Wallace Tower 1280, Houston, TX 77030, USA;
[b] Shirley Ryan Ability Lab, Northwestern Fienberg School of Medicine, 345 East Superior Street, Chicago, IL 60611, USA
* Corresponding author.
E-mail address: fabiola.i.reyes@gmail.com

Phys Med Rehabil Clin N Am 31 (2020) 117–129
https://doi.org/10.1016/j.pmr.2019.09.002

people with cerebral palsy (CP) benefit from many of these applications. Currently, technology is being used to enhance mobility, provide assistance with activities of daily living (ADLs), optimize communication, and improve education.

The use of technology and its application for neurorehabilitation is in part based on the theory of neuroplasticity, the restoration of neural networks through behavioral training.[4] Technology can also be used to make rote exercises more engaging. The affordability and wide use of smart phones and tablets has created equalizing opportunities for our patients and families[5] by making rehabilitation tools more accessible.

This article provides an overview on how technology is used to address mobility, self-care, communication, and motivation to maximize rehabilitation in individuals affected by CP. The role that technology plays in educating patients, families, and health care providers is also discussed.

MOBILITY ROBOTICS

The field of robotics is broadly defined as a branch of technology that deals with the design and integration of robots and computer systems to help perform human tasks by providing control, sensory feedback and information processing.[6] In the field of neurorehabilitation, the principles of motor learning and neuroplasticity can be applied with the intent of improving quality of movement. Neuroplasticity relies on high-intensity, repetitive patterns to enhance function[4] and robots can be designed to provide high doses of guided movements.[7,8] Robots can also support joints, provide resistance or assistance, and provide real-time feedback.[4,9] The ability to manipulate robot parameters can allow a patient to exert more effort gradually and robots can quantify effort.[10]

Mobility robots can be categorized by describing the design or functional task it helps to achieve.[3] Functional classification can be based on whether the device augments or assists functional movements, and whether these movements target the upper or lower extremity. Engineering texts often categorize rehabilitation robots based on design: grounded exoskeletons, wearable exoskeletons, and end effector devices. Exoskeletons in general have the ability to control individual joints, whereas end effector devices control limb segments and can provide a wider range of resistive and assistive forces on the limb.

The use of robotics to address mobility in individuals with CP, and specifically children, has been adopted relatively recently compared with its adaption into other rehabilitation fields, such as rehabilitation in adults who have had strokes.[11] Publications addressing the use of robotics in rehabilitation of children with CP have grown at a remarkable rate.[2] Two primary concerns found in the literature are choice of outcome measures and apparatus size. Although many studies focus on body structure and movement, a lack of focus on patient-related tasks limits the evaluation of how rehabilitation robots impact activities and participation.[12] Currently, most of the mobility robots available in the market are sized for adults.

Gait Training Robotics

Treadmill training that integrates grounded exoskeleton designs and partial body weight supported training has grown rapidly in last few decades. This type of augmentative assistive robotic device provides simulation of the gait cycle as well as visual and auditory feedback to improve gait quality and efficiency.[13]

Although treadmill training has been rapidly adopted in many rehabilitation settings, currently only a few randomized controlled studies have been conducted and evidence to determine its effectiveness in the rehabilitation of people affected by CP is still lacking. A systematic review published by Carvalho and colleagues[14] in 2017 identified 10 studies that addressed gait training with robotic therapy in people with CP. A meta-analysis suggested that robotic gait training improves gait walking speed, endurance, and motor function, especially among people with CP classified as Gross Motor Function Classification System (GMFCS) levels I and II. Despite the encouraging findings, a cause and effect relationship could not be established between robotic gait training and improvement in gait function.[14] The lack of established rehabilitation protocols and the diversity of study settings make it difficult for aggregate studies to achieve sufficient power. Thus, the efficacy of gait training robots has yet to be established.[1] Given these challenges, experts in rehabilitation robotics have called for standardized protocols so that quality information can be gathered with the goal of advancing rehabilitation robotic technology.[1]

Lower Extremity Robotics

Robotics that target motion at a joint typically use end effector and grounded exoskeleton designs to provide movement with more than 1° of freedom. In the field of rehabilitation of children with CP, this technology can be used to help address specific joint and muscle characteristics, such as joint range of motion, muscle strength, muscle length, and spasticity.[15,16] Ankle robotics have been the most frequently studied.[17] These robots can be paired with task specific games to target movements and have the ability to provide passive, active-assistive, active, and active-resistive exercises.[18] Measures that have been used to study these types of robotics include active and passive range of motion, strength, selective motor control, as well as activity measures such as climbing stairs, balance, and walking distances. Incorporating ankle robotics into clinical practice is feasible. Therapists' knowledge, preference, and goals of therapy all need to be taken into consideration. Some devices have the potential to be used in the home, so rehabilitation can extend beyond the walls of the clinic.[19,20]

Upper Extremity Robotics

Because joint movements in the upper extremity are complex, careful consideration of joint alignment must be applied in upper extremity robotic design. Studies that apply the use of upper extremity robotics have looked at outcome measures that address both quality of movement and functional tasks. Quality of movement measures can include range of motion, muscle tone, and kinematics such as upper extremity speed, aim, deviation from target, and smoothness of movement. The Fugl-Myer Assessment is an example of a functional measure used in the literature.[11] The use of robots to improve function of the upper extremities is promising; however, sufficient high-quality evidence is still lacking and effectiveness in this patient has not been established.

Wearable Exoskeletons

These robotic devices are wearable units that incorporate motors, pneumatics, levers, and hydraulics and are controlled by a microprocessor and powered by batteries with the purpose of supporting movements.[21] Most current designs target gait efficiency. Compared with grounded exoskeletons, wearable exoskeletons are more portable and have the potential to be used in settings outside of the clinical environment. Initially, this type of robotic device was designed for the rehabilitation of individuals with spinal cord injuries, and clinical effectiveness has mostly been tested on this patient population.[21–23] Benefits of exoskeleton use in the spinal chord injury population reported in the literature include improved mobility, decreased spasticity, and improved bowel regularity.[23]

Based on existing technology, new designs have focused on adapting wearable exoskeletons to address mobility in other populations, such as in individuals affected by CP. Design considerations for this patient population include size, portability, and use of light weight materials.[22] Currently, most of the studies that address rehabilitation of children with CP in the literature have limited sample size, or are feasibility studies that use exoskeletons in the lower extremities to address specific gait patterns in ambulatory children.[24,25]

Well-designed clinical studies are needed to establish the safety and efficacy of exoskeletons in children with CP. Some safety issues to consider are risks of pressure sores, fractures and falls, as well as time burden of fitting the device.[21]

VIRTUAL REALITY SYSTEMS

Virtual reality systems use interactive, real-time simulations by integrating computer software and hardware into a user–computer interface to promote multi-sensory stimulation and user interaction.[26] It has been proposed that virtual reality experiences integrate 4 basic concepts to make an experience more real: immersion-the presentation of sensory cues; interaction, - visual, tactile and auditory feedback that allows users to self-identify with the visual body; sensorimotor contingencies-the response of the virtual environment to the actions of the user; and illusions-the perception of physical presence in an alternate or imaged world or environment.[26]

Virtual Reality Technologies for Motor Learning

Sensorimotor training with virtual reality technologies is in theory achieved by engaging motor and perceptual areas of the brain through the provision of multisensory body related feedback in real time.[27] Virtual reality systems can allow the user to practice good quality movements and high number of repetitions by simulating a real-life task.[28] For motor learning, virtual reality systems can help target functional movements of the whole body or individual limbs.[28] The designs and availability of the virtual reality systems that have been studied vary widely. Some studies, for example, use interactive commercial video games and others use engineered technology that is customized and incorporates real-time movement analysis and feedback.[29,30]

A meta-analysis by Chen and colleagues[30] in 2018 looked at research conducted in the field of motor rehabilitation of children with CP and analyzed 19 studies that used virtual reality interventions. Most studies targeted gait, upper extremity movement, and balance. The review suggested that virtual reality had a medium to large effect on the rehabilitation of gait and large effect on the rehabilitation of balance. Engineered virtual reality systems that target the upper extremity showed greater positive effect in improving function than commercially available systems.

When the outcomes in the review were broken down into categories by the International Classification of Disease model, virtual reality interventions were found to have a large effect by activity component, medium effect by body structure and function component, and a small effect based on participation component. The heterogeneity of study participants and study protocols were cited as factors affecting the quality of overall evidence.

Although virtual reality is showing some promise, the degree of immersion can be quite variable, and experts in the engineering field have proposed that interactive games should not be considered an equal technology to immersive technologies when studying neurorehabilitation outcomes.[26]

AUGMENTATIVE AND ALTERNATIVE COMMUNICATION SYSTEMS

It is estimated that up to 40% of children with CP classified as GMFCS levels IV and V have some difficulties with communication[31]. In addition, up to 50% of children with CP who could benefit from augmentative and alternative communication (AAC) systems are not receiving services to address this.[32] Reasons cited for the gap in the use of AAC include lack of access to technology and delays in identification of language problems early in life.[32] Factors that affect communication in children with CP vary widely because the heterogeneity of the condition can affect many aspects of communication.[32] Even after an individual with communication difficulties has been identified as a candidate for AAC, finding the correct communication device can take time and multiple trials. Once the correct device is identified, effectiveness depends on the user's motivation, communication partners, social context, and the purpose of interaction.[33]

Communication aide designs can range from manual signs and graphic symbols to more complex devices that generate speech.[33] Recent technological gains have yielded light weight, cost-effective, and accurate input sensors for devices that generate speech.[31] This development has made it easier to incorporate different types of user interfaces onto AAC devices and addresses the needs of people with varying degrees of physical abilities. More recently, designs have integrated communication aides with other technological devices, such as those that can also allow the user to operate their mobile phone, browse the Internet, or operate home devices.[34]

Complex AAC devices are typically made up of 3 components: an access pathway, a signal processing unit, and an alternative communication system.[31,35] The access pathway can be designed so that information can be entered in a variety of ways. Inputs, for example, can be controlled with axial, appendicular, or eye movements. After the message is entered, the signal processing unit, which is usually a microcontroller, manipulates the information so that it can be converted into an output. The alternative communication system provides the output, which can be in the form of verbal or written communicaiton.[36] Verbal outputs can be prefabricated or put together by the user or his caregivers. Text output requires reading abilities in both the sender and receiver of communication.

AAC devices can capture the message to be delivered by the sender in a variety of ways. Letter-based systems are usually slower and require a specific level of literacy,[33] whereas icon-based systems are faster but can be more ambiguous.[36] Information input can also be either direct or indirect.[31] For direct systems, the user selects the letter or icon from choices presented in a linear or grid system. This allows the user to provide the pace of information selection. Indirect methods of information selection are system paced, because the user has to wait for a letter or icon to appear before he chooses it.[35]

Augmentative and Alternative Communication Devices with Active Inputs

Inputs requiring eye gaze control
People with reliable eye movements can communicate information through an access pathway that is controlled with eye gaze.[37] Eye gaze captures eye movement through an infrared camera mounted on a computer or a tablet.[37] The infrared camera allows the user to move a cursor on the computer. Letters or pictures can then be selected by holding the eye gaze on a specific object or letter or by blinking. To allow for accurate selection and promote ergonomic posture, the access pathway must be mounted for optimal recognition of eye movements.

Inputs requiring controlled movements

Owing to the heterogeneity of motor impairments associated with CP, a wide range of setups can be configured into the access pathway. These user interfaces can be specifically chosen to accommodate gross motor or fine motor control limitations. User interfaces can include standard designs such as trackballs, joystick, mice, and keyboards.[31] Adapted setups that take into account greater motor impairments described in the literature include mechanical switches, head control inputs, and adapted jackets.[31,35] For those for whom motor control makes axial and appendicular movements especially difficult, access pathways can be set up so that mouth movements, tongue movements, and intraoral air pressure can be used to enter information.[31]

Augmentative and Alternative Communication Devices with Passive Inputs

Physiologic inputs

For individuals who may not be able to initiate volitional movements, access pathways may have the potential to decode signs or clues that indicate feelings or needs.[31] For example, studies have looked at vital signs and facial expressions to communicate emotional state. Accelerometers may also be able to decode movements in dyskinetic children to detect intention. AAC technology that uses physiologic inputs to communicate implied intent is still in its infancy and most studies are in the early phases of design. Studying these devices may also be difficult as studying accuracy of communication in individuals with very limited volitional movements may not be able to verify the accuracy of the communication output.

Brain–computer interface

CP advocacy groups have recently identified AAC technology that can potentially convert thoughts into speech as a priority in technological research and development.[38] Brain–computer interfaces are able to detect thought-induced changes in the brain and convert this information in a processing unit to produce communication output. Brain–computer interfaces were initially invasive and required electrodes to be placed directly onto the brain. More recent technology has allowed the electroencephalograph to be used to capture information input. Early designs of brain–computer interfaces used imagery to control hardware to perform movements, such as grabbing objects with a robotic arm.[39] The brain–computer interface has recently incorporated icon and letter-based access pathways to produce speech for those whose head, neck, and eye movements are limited or cause too much fatigue.[36] Although the development of the brain–computer interface is a priority to enhance the function of those with CP,[37] research studies in this population are still limited.[39]

Augmentative and Alternative Communication Device Benefits

AAC devices benefit individuals with CP because they allow for communication independence, improved interactions with peers, more involvement in self-care, and better means to assess cognition and development.[31] Other benefits noted in studies include increased interactions with others, improved ability to make choices and to do school schoolwork, ease of care giver burden, and improved psychological well-being[37,40,41]

Augmentative and Alternative Communication Device Limitations

Similar to other technologies, the use of the AAC does not come without drawbacks. First, these devices can be expensive, and the cost of training the user to be an effective communication sender should also be considered. Device abandonment,[42] durability and service requirements have also been noted as limiting factors associated with AAC devices.[43] Portability and size of the devices should also be considered. Finally, AAC devices provide a much slower means of communication. Typical verbal speech produces150 to 250 words per minute, whereas it is estimated that AAC devices produce about 2 to 15 words per minute.[44] Slow language output can thus make AAC use frustrating for both the sender and receiver of communication.

SELF-CARE AND SOCIAL ROBOTS

The design and study of robots to assist people with care has grown rapidly since the early 2000s.[45] Because health care robots can be used for physical support, social support, and health care monitoring, many robotic systems have been conceptualized with the intent of aiding older adults.[46] Robots used to help with physical tasks associated with self-care and socialization have the potential to promote independence in people with CP.

Activities of Daily Living Robots

Personal care robots that help with ADLs can be especially helpful for adults with CP who have limited use of the upper extremities. These robots have been described in the literature as systems containing a manipulator with at least 3° of freedom that allow the robotic device to perform every day activities through interactions with the user.[45] They can be designed as mounted devices that are placed on a surface such as a table, desk, or lap tray, or as autonomous robotic systems with driving and navigation capabilities. The user interface can include keyboards, joysticks, keypads, switches, touch screens, voice recognition, gesture recognition, and buttons.[45]

An example of a robot that has been studied is one that can obtain liquids for consumption while simultaneously navigating thin corridors and avoiding obstacles.[47] Other task specific robots have been studied using a wheelchair-mounted devices, and include robots that can grasp a bottle, push calculator buttons, and pour water from a bottle.[48] More specific ADL tasks studied have looked at brushing teeth, eating, and face washing.[49] Robots used to aid feeding have also been developed,[50] and the literature on these robots has focused on fine-tuning movements and correcting mistakes.[51] Overall, ease of use and perceived safety have been demonstrated in the literature,[45] but there is still a gap in studies that look into the applicability of this technology for the benefit of individuals with CP.

Similar to AAC devices, many factors should be considered in selecting an ADL robot. Specifically, for children and adults with CP, a lack of motor control may make it more difficult to manipulate touch screens, joysticks, or keyboards. Larger, more sensitive buttons may work better for this population. In addition, the ability to mount a user interface for access and manipulation may also be an important consideration. Training and portability of the device should also be addressed, because these factors can influence device abandonment.[52]

Although robots designed to help with self-care have been launched into the market, prototypes are also being researched in academic facilities. One research approach is to study general purpose robots and their ability to be programmed to assist with ADLs. The Robots for Humanity Project is one such approach. This project uses mobile robots that physically manipulate the environment to provide assistance to people with disabilities.[53] The group is meshing user-centered design, shared autonomy (with the robot) principles, and user interface optimization to enhance the quality of life of individuals with motor impairments. Although this project started with designs to address independence in an adult with quadriplegia owing to a brainstem stroke, these same concepts have the potential to be expanded for use by children and adults with CP.

Social Robots

Socially assistive robots focus on helping users via noncontact interactions to engage them in social interactions.[54] These type of robots can be used a tool to provide tutoring, physical therapy instruction, or planning of daily activities. They can also provide a means of emotional expression for individuals with cognitive, physical, communication, or social impairments.

Social robots that help conduct therapy programs are currently being studied in children with CP. These socially assistive robots help maximize therapy sessions by providing motivation and instruction.[55,56] They provide motivation with phrases and stories and provide physical demonstration of exercises to instruct children during therapy sessions.[56] In some cases, the use of socially assistive robots can be integrated with other technologies, such as virtual reality. Social robots have the potential to be useful tools in the area of CP rehabilitation, however, most studies currently only address technical development and feasibility of use.[57] Experimental studies that incorporate social robots into rehabilitation programs and measure functional outcomes are still lacking.[55] In future studies, it will also be important to consider the acceptance of social assistive robots by the health care team.[46]

MOBILE APPLICATIONS

It is estimated that worldwide, 36% of the population uses a smartphone. Mobile phone accessibility, in part, has prompted the rapid developmental of mobile applications (apps) to address health care needs.[58] Owing to the rapid development of this technology and the wide breadth of needs that apps can cover, the mobile application trends described in this article are meant to give an overview of how these applications can be used to maximize the care and rehabilitation of people with CP. Given the breadth of apps that are available, websites that categorize, describe, and provide access to applications for individuals with CP can be particularly useful to families, health providers and educators. One example of such a web site is the BridgingApps web page, which was designed to bridge the gap between technology and people with disabilities.[59]

CP related mobile apps can be broken down into 3 main categories: general applications that can address the health and mobility of patients with CP, CP-specific applications intended for use by patients and their families, and CP-specific application intended for use by health care providers. Although there are many applications available on many different platforms, studies that look at the usefulness of these apps are much more limited, with most studies looking at the usefulness of applications that provide assessment tools meant for use for health care providers.[60]

General Mobile Applications

Examples of general platforms that can be used for health care management include apps that help organize medical and therapy history, apps that provide education on healthy habits and general well-being, apps that provide information about legislative updates and resources, and apps that provide games and advice to help promote motor milestone development.[60] General mobility and accessibility apps can also be used by individuals with CP and provide maps with information about public transportation accessibility, information about accessible parking, and ride sharing programs that can help users find/hail vehicles with capabilities to accommodate different mobility equipment.

Cerebral Palsy-Specific Mobile Applications for Patients and Their Families

Apps intended specifically for people with CP and their families can help guide motor, linguistic and cognitive exercises. There are also specific CP applications that can help users organize medical information and therapies. Some apps provide education and information that is specific to the diagnosis of CP. Apps that can provide AAC through tablets or mobile phones have also been able to make AAC more accessible to users that may otherwise not have the means to acquire more complex devices.[31] The CP Channel developed by the Cerebral Palsy Foundation is unique in that it has international experts on CP providing age-based and function-based learning topics for the convenience of parents, children, teenagers, and adults. This type of platform provides vetted material that equalizes learning and allows for personalized content.[61]

Cerebral Palsy-Specific Mobile Applications for Health Care Providers

Apps used by health care providers include those that help to characterize motor movements, provide directed therapy and exercises, and provide tools and risk calculations for musculoskeletal disorders such as hip subluxation. Professional groups now also have more and more access to sharing of ideas, updates, and policies through social media groups, which are often accessed through apps. Professional organizations such as the American Academy of Cerebral Palsy and Developmental Medicine are now using applications to help national conference attendees organize their schedules and access lectures.

SUMMARY

It is an exciting time in the field of rehabilitation, because rapid technological advances provide new and innovative means of extending rehabilitation and education to people with CP and their families. Although rehabilitation technologies have the potential to provide more individualized, dose-intensive, and engaging rehabilitation, many factors should be taken into consideration in the design of these technologies. Teams of stakeholders including clinicians, engineers, researchers and developers should be created to ensure that rehabilitation technologies are being used to improve not only body function and structure, but also activities and participation. Effective training strategies and easy to use designs should also be incorporated to avoid device abandonment. Moving forward, it will be important to ensure that technologies are being defined appropriately to prevent confounding research results. In addition, prioritizing sound methodology and meaningful and consistent outcome measures will be of utmost importance when designing studies to test the efficacy of these technologies. We must also perform careful cost–benefit analyses to ensure fiscal responsibility to individuals with CP and their families. Because most health information is now digitized, ensuring the privacy of our patient's health information should be a high priority when designing, testing, and using technology in the rehabilitation setting.

When recommending a technology, we, as physical medicine and rehabilitation specialists are ensuring the safety and efficacy of an innovation. The feasibility and safety of each technology needs testing before it is implemented. Technology can open worlds in communication, mobility, and independence in ADLs and learning. Our specialty is unique in that we focus on function, and can play an active role in the technological revolution by assisting on input for design of devices and research, trialing patient populations, and advocating for medical necessity when appropriate for children and adults with CP.

REFERENCES

1. Van Hedel HJA, Severini G, Scarton A, et al. Advanced Robotic Therapy Integrated Centers (ARTIC): an international collaboration facilitating the application of rehabilitation technologies. J Neuroeng Rehabil 2018;15(1):1–16.
2. Krebs HI, Volpe BT. Rehabilitation robotics. Handb Clin Neurol 2013;110:283–94.
3. Gassert R, Dietz V. Rehabilitation robots for the treatment of sensorimotor deficits: a neurophysiological perspective. J Neuroeng Rehabil 2018;15(1):1–15.
4. Kleim JA, Jones TA. Principles of experience-dependent neural plasticity: implications for rehabilitation after brain damage. J Speech Lang Hear Res 2008; 51(1):S225.
5. Anderson KM, Olson S. Roundtable on the promotion of health equity and the elimination of health disparities. Washington, DC: Board on Population Health and Public Health Practice; Health and Medicine Division; National Academies of Sciences, Engineering, and Medicine; 2016. The Promises and Perils.
6. Tirgul CS, Naik MR. Artificial intelligence and robots. Int J Adv Res Comput Eng Technol 2016;5(6):1278–323.
7. Islam MR, Spiewak C, Rahman MH, et al. A brief review on robotic exoskeletons for upper extremity rehabilitation to find the gap between research porotype and commercial type. Adv Robot Autom 2017;06(03):1–12.
8. Wallard L, Dietrich G, Kerlirzin Y, et al. Effect of robotic-assisted gait rehabilitation on dynamic equilibrium control in the gait of children with cerebral palsy. Gait Posture 2018;60:55–60.
9. Riener R, Frey M, Bernhardt M, et al. Human-centered rehabilitation robotics. 2005 IEEE International Conference on Rehabilitation Robotics (ICORR), Chicago 2005. p. 319–22.
10. Ross SA, Foreman M, Engsberg JR. Comparison of 3 different methods to analyze ankle plantarflexor stiffness in children with spastic diplegia cerebral palsy. Arch Phys Med Rehabil 2011;92(12):2034–40.
11. Chen YP, Howard AM. Effects of robotic therapy on upper-extremity function in children with cerebral palsy: a systematic review. Dev Neurorehabil 2016;19(1): 64–71.
12. Katelaar M, Vermeer A, Hart H. Effects of a functional therapy children with cerebral palsy. Phys Ther 2001;81:1534–45.
13. Bayon C, Raya R. Robotic therapies for children with cerebral palsy: a systematic review. Transl Biomed 2016;7(1):1–10.
14. Carvalho I, Pinto SM, Chagas D, et al. Robotic gait training for individuals with cerebral palsy: a systematic review and meta-analysis. Arch Phys Med Rehabil 2017;98(11):2332–44.
15. Sukal-Moulton T, Clancy T, Zhang LQ, et al. Clinical application of a robotic ankle training program for cerebral palsy compared to the research laboratory application: does it translate to practice? Arch Phys Med Rehabil 2014;95(8):1433–40.
16. Wu YN, Hwang M, Ren Y, et al. Combined passive stretching and active movement rehabilitation of lower-limb impairments in children with cerebral palsy using a portable robot. Neurorehabil Neural Repair 2011;25(4):378–85.
17. Zhang M, Daview TC, Xie S. Effectiveness of robot-assisted therapy on ankle rehabilitation–a systematic review. J Neuroeng Rehabil 2013;10:30.

18. Krebs HI, Palazzolo JJ, Dipietro L, et al. Rehabilitation robotics: performance-based progressive robot-assisted therapy. Auton Robots 2003;15(7):20.

19. Chen K, Member I, Ren Y, et al. Home - based tele - assisted robotic rehabilitation of joint impairments in children with cerebral palsy. Conf Proc IEEE Eng Med Biol Soc 2014;2014:5288–91.

20. Lang CE, MacDonald JR, Gnip C. Counting repetitions: an observational study of outpatient therapy for people with hemiparesis post-stroke. J Neurol Phys Ther 2007;31(1):3–10.

21. Gorgey AS. Robotic exoskeletons: the current pros and cons. World J Orthop 2018;9(9):112–9.

22. Burton A. Expecting exoskeletons for more than spinal cord injury. Lancet Neurol 2018;17(4):302–3.

23. Miller LE, Zimmermann AK, Herbert WG. Clinical effectiveness and safety of powered exoskeleton-assisted walking in patients with spinal cord injury: systematic review with meta-analysis. Med Devices (Auckl) 2016;9:455–66.

24. Lerner ZF, Damiano DL, Bulea TC. The effects of exoskeleton assisted knee extension on lower-extremity gait kinematics, kinetics, and muscle activity in children with cerebral palsy. Sci Rep 2017;7(1):1–12.

25. Lerner ZF, Harvey TA, Lawson JL. A battery-powered ankle exoskeleton improves gait mechanics in a feasibility study of individuals with cerebral palsy. Ann Biomed Eng 2019;47(6):1345–56.

26. Perez-Marcos D. Virtual reality experiences, embodiment, videogames and their dimensions in neurorehabilitation. J Neuroeng Rehabil 2018;15(1):113.

27. Adamovich SV, Fluet GG, Tunik E, et al. Sensorimotor training in virtual reality: a review. NeuroRehabilitation 2009;25(1):29–44.

28. Galvin J, Levac D. Facilitating clinical decision-making about the use of virtual reality within paediatric motor rehabilitation: describing and classifying virtual reality systems. Dev Neurorehabil 2011;14(2):112–22.

29. Booth ATC, Buizer AI, Harlaar J, et al. Immediate effects of immersive biofeedback on gait in children with cerebral pals. Arch Phys Med Rehabil 2018; 100(4):598–605.

30. Chen YP, Fanchiang H, Howard AM. Effectiveness of virtual reality in children with cerebral palsy: a systematic review and meta-analysis of randomized controlled trials. Phys Ther 2018;98(1):63–77.

31. Myrden A, Schudlo L, Weyand S, et al. Trends in communicative access solutions for children with cerebral palsy. J Child Neurol 2014;29(8):1108–18.

32. Smith AL, Hustad KC. AAC and early intervention for children with cerebral palsy: parent perceptions and child risk factors. Augment Altern Commun 2015;31(4): 336–50.

33. Light J, Drager K. AAC technologies for young children with complex communication needs: state of the science and future research directions. Augment Altern Commun 2007;23(3):204–16.

34. Morin KL, Ganz JB, Gregori EV, et al. A systematic quality review of high-tech AAC interventions as an evidence-based practice. Augment Altern Commun 2018;34(2):104–17.

35. Lampe R, Blumenstein T, Turova V, et al. Mobile communication jacket for people with severe speech impairment. Disabil Rehabil Assist Technol 2018;13(3):280–6.

36. Ahani A, Moghadamfalahi M, Erdogmus D. Language-model assisted and icon-based communication through a brain-computer interface with different presentation paradigms. IEEE Trans Neural Syst Rehabil Eng 2018;26(9):1835–44.

37. Karlsson P, Allsop A, Dee-Price BJ, et al. Eye-gaze control technology for children, adolescents and adults with cerebral palsy with significant physical disability: findings from a systematic review. Dev Neurorehabil 2018;21(8): 497–505.

38. Cerebral Palsy Alliance. Advancing innovation in assistive technology summit 2018; San Francisco, May 3-4, 2018. Available at: https://cerebralpalsy.org.au/wp-content/uploads/2019/05/7_2018_A-summary-of-the-Advancing-Innovation-in-Assistive-Technology-Summit-2018_10_September_2018_Final.pdf. Accessed March 13, 2019.

39. Zhang J, Jadavji Z, Zewdie E, et al. Evaluating if children can use simple brain computer interfaces. Front Hum Neurosci 2019;13:1–7.

40. Borgestig M, Sandqvist J, Falkmer T, et al. Gaze-based assistive technology in daily activities in children with severe physical impairments–an intervention study. Dev Neurorehabil 2016;20(3):129–41.

41. Hwang C-S, Weng H-H, Chang H-T, et al. An eye-tracking assistive device improves the quality of life for ALS patients and reduces the caregivers' burden. J Mot Behav 2014;46(4):233–8.

42. Johnson JM, Inglebret E, Jones C, et al. Perspectives of speech language pathologists regarding success versus abandonment of AAC. Augment Altern Commun 2006;22(2):85–99.

43. Karlsson P, Johnston C, Barker K. Influences on students' assistive technology use at school: the views of classroom teachers, allied health professionals, students with cerebral palsy and their parents. Disabil Rehabil Assist Technol 2018;13(8):763–71.

44. Bertucco M, Sanger TD. A model to estimate the optimal layout for assistive communication touchscreen devices in children with dyskinetic cerebral palsy. IEEE Trans Neural Syst Rehabil Eng 2018;26(7):1371–80.

45. Bilyea A, Seth N, Nesathurai S, et al. Robotic assistants in personal care: a scoping review. Med Eng Phys 2017;49(2017):1–6.

46. Hall AK, Sung M, Backonja U, et al. Acceptance and perceived usefulness of robots to assist with activities of daily living and healthcare tasks. Assist Technol 2019;31(3):133–40.

47. Jacobs T, Graf B. Practical evaluation of service robots for support and routine tasks in an elderly care facility. 2012 IEEE Workshop on Advanced Robotics and its Social Impacts (ARSO), Munich 2012. pp. 46–49.

48. Maheu V, Archambault PS, Frappier J, et al. Evaluation of the JACO robotic arm: clinico-economic study for powered wheelchair users with upper-extremity disabilities. IEEE Int Conf Rehabil Robot 2011;2011:5975397.

49. Jardón A, Gil ÁM, De La Peña AI, et al. Usability assessment of ASIBOT: a portable robot to aid patients with spinal cord injury. Disabil Rehabil Assist Technol 2011;6(4):320–30.

50. Park D, Kim YK, Erickson ZM, et al. Towards assistive feeding with a generalpurpose mobile manipulator. 2016 ICRA Workshop on Human-Robot Interfaces for Enhanced Physical Interactions (ICRA), Stockholm 2016. pp. 3–6.

51. Park D, Kim H, Kemp CC. Multimodal anomaly detection for assistive robots. Auton Robots 2018;43(3):611–29.

52. Phillips B, Zhao H. Predictors of assistive technology abandonment. Assist Technol 1993;5(1):36–45.

53. Chen TL, Ciocarlie M, Cousins S, et al. Robots for humanity: using assistive robotics to empower people with disabilities. IEEE Robot Autom Mag 2013; 20(1):30–9.

54. Feil-Seifer D, Matarić MJ. Defining socially assistive robotics. Proc 2005 IEEE 9th Int Conf Rehabil Robot 2005;2005:465–8.
55. Psychouli P, Cheng P, Dimopoulos C. Development of a robotic system for enhancing children's motivation and constraint induced movement therapy (CIMT). Stud Health Technol Inform 2017;242:479–83.
56. Carillo MF, Butchart J, Knight S, et al. Adapting a general purpose social robot for paediatric rehabilitation through in-situ design. ACM Trans Human-Robot Interact 2018;7:3–30.
57. Dawe J, Sutherland C, Barco A, et al. Can social robots help children in health-care contexts? A scoping review. BMJ Paediatr Open 2019;3(1):e000371.
58. Qudah B, Luetsch K. The influence of mobile health applications on patient -healthcare provider relationships: a systematic, narrative review. Patient Educ Couns 2019.
59. BridgingApps. Available at: https://www.bridgingapps.org/. Accessed May 24, 2019.
60. Rodriguez Mariblanca M, Cano De la Cuerda R. Aplicacinoes moviles en la par-alisis cerebral infantil. Neurologia 2017.
61. CP channel. Cerebral Palsy Foundation. Available at: https://www.yourcpf.org/cpproduct/cp-channel/. Accessed March 13, 2019.

Outcome Assessment and Function in Cerebral Palsy

Jilda N. Vargus-Adams, MD, MSc[a,b,c,*]

KEYWORDS

- Cerebral palsy • Function • Outcome measure • Outcomes • Disability

KEY POINTS

- Challenges to outcome measurement in CP include the breadth and variability of CP, the chronicity of concerns, and a mismatch of disability with a medical model.
- Current outcome measures can be best understood using the International Classification of Functioning, Disability and Health as framework.
- Careful selection of outcome measures informs clinical care and research.

INTRODUCTION

Care and research in childhood cerebral palsy (CP) continue to evolve. As understanding of CP grows more nuanced, so grows interest in describing the status of children with CP—their function, their activities, their challenges, and their adaptations. Outcome measurement is the way the status of patients and research subjects is described, including the many ways they function. Outcomes include any parameters of human existence from blood pressure to walking speed to quality of life. The tools used to measure outcomes may be laboratory tests, physical examinations, questionnaires, interviews, or any other evaluations. These tools may be called outcome measures, instruments, or assessments. In CP, outcome measurement is of great significance because having robust means of measuring outcomes is vital to understanding the utility of treatments. Research must first accurately measure the things that matter for children with CP, for without that reliable ruler, it cannot be established if interventions are having useful effects. This article addresses the challenges of outcome measurement in CP, the current status of outcome measurement in CP, and the issues of understanding change in childhood CP.

[a] Department of Pediatrics, University of Cincinnati College of Medicine, Cincinnati, OH, USA;
[b] Department of Neurology and Rehabilitation Medicine, University of Cincinnati College of Medicine, Cincinnati, OH, USA; [c] Division of Pediatric Rehabilitation Medicine, Cincinnati Children's Hospital Medical Center, 3333 Burnet Avenue, MLC-4009, Cincinnati, OH 45229-3039, USA
* Division of Pediatric Rehabilitation Medicine, Cincinnati Children's Hospital Medical Center, 3333 Burnet Avenue, MLC-4009, Cincinnati, OH 45229-3039.
E-mail address: Jilda.Vargus-Adams@cchmc.org

Phys Med Rehabil Clin N Am 31 (2020) 131–141
https://doi.org/10.1016/j.pmr.2019.09.011
1047-9651/20/© 2019 Elsevier Inc. All rights reserved.

pmr.theclinics.com

MEASUREMENT CHALLENGES WITH CEREBRAL PALSY

Outcome measurement in children with CP presents an array of challenges. The issues of concern for children with CP are wide ranging, chronic, difficult to quantify, resistant to change, and more reflective of disability than illness. These parameters may frustrate the clinician or researcher who wishes to evaluate the status of a child or youth with CP.

Breadth

As any person with CP, parent, or medical professional who cares for children with CP will attest, CP touches almost every aspect of life. CP causes changes in basic body functioning, such as strength, coordination, and muscle tone. CP results in difficulty with functional tasks like swallowing, walking, dressing, and communicating. In turn, these deficits may contribute to decreased involvement in community, school, and family activities. CP has some impact on quality of life[1] and definitely creates additional stressors for caregivers.[2] Thus, there are many potential problem areas to understand and to measure in CP. The sheer number of possible targets for measurement means that describing CP in a comprehensive and accurate way often is difficult to do.

Variability

Secondly, CP is a diverse diagnosis with substantial variation in impairments and severity. Although CP may manifest with marked impairments and myriad secondary impacts, some individuals with CP have fairly modest disability and relatively few daily effects. Furthermore, CP is highly associated with other conditions, including intellectual disability and seizures that create their own issues. Because of the variability in symptoms, sequelae, and comorbidities, the concepts that are of concern may vary greatly between children. Depending on the unique status of each child or youth with CP, a meaningful evaluation may include different outcome measures if the evaluation is targeted to the issues affecting each individual. These differences create a need for flexibility in measurement strategies so as to address each child with CP in a productive fashion.

Chronicity

Another challenge is the long-term nature of CP. CP is not an acute illness. Children and youth with CP will always have CP, but their CP may have an impact on them differently over time. It is of paramount importance to understand the long-term outcomes of CP and how interventions affect outcomes many years later. Studying outcomes in a longitudinal fashion over years, rather than weeks or months, is expensive, time consuming, and messy due to the inability to control for extraneous factors. Nonetheless, longitudinal measurements are arguably the most important means to explore treatments and interventions for CP, because outcomes in adolescence and adulthood are of critical importance.

No Benchmarks

There are few gold standards or rubrics for measurement in CP. Many of the domains of concern are not easily quantified and there are no established benchmarks of measurement. For example, even in terms of walking, there is no single, best, and universally accepted method to measure how well a child with CP walks. Assessing concepts like quality of movement, happiness, ease of care, and independence is a confusing and frustrating venture. Unlike more quantifiable outcomes (temperature or birth weight, for example), many concerns in CP do not have an established ruler to measure them.

Stasis

One goal of outcome measurement is to assess changes that occur as a result of treatments or interventions. This is a particular challenge in CP because many of the available treatments do not seem to create big changes. With small treatment effects described or anticipated for many interventions, ambiguity can arise over the quality of the available outcome measurements. If the change is real, should not a really good measure be able to show the change? Imagine a situation where an outcome measure is used before and after a treatment in order to see if the treatment is effective. If the score on the measure does not change, 2 conclusions might be reached: either the measurement tool is not adequately sensitive to change and cannot detect meaningful effects of treatment or the treatment has insufficient effect to be meritorious. Until each individual outcome measure can be evaluated for its discriminatory properties and responsiveness to change, this conundrum will remain.

Medical Model Mismatch

A final challenge in measurement in CP is the difficulty of looking at CP with a purely medical perspective. This perspective considers CP to be a disease and people with CP to be ill. It suggests that CP is something that has clear biological markers and that medical interventions can or should be used to alter the underlying disease process. These ideas translate into a measurement paradigm that includes an assumption that the basic processes of CP should be targeted with treatments and that improving the physiologic parameters of CP will result in improvements in the outcomes of interest. Generally, this is how things are considered for most health conditions. In cases of CP, however, this approach is not entirely satisfactory. First of all, many people with CP are not ill and are best described as having a disability rather than as being in poor health. When viewed as a chronic disability, CP is not something that is amenable to direct treatment. Furthermore, the degree of impairment in the more basic issues of CP (like spasticity or strength) does not directly translate into functional (dis)abilities or more higher-level issues like quality of life. Thus, some of the typical assumptions about health-related outcome measurement are not fully applicable in CP. Understanding issues like change, individual preferences and goals, or the role of societal constructs in CP becomes even more salient when CP is viewed as a disability.

STATE OF PRACTICE IN CEREBRAL PALSY OUTCOMES
The International Classification of Functioning, Disability and Health as a Framework

In the past 10 years, perspectives on outcome assessment in CP have been influenced and shaped by the World Health Organization International Classification of Functioning, Disability and Health (ICF)[3] as a guiding principle. This seminal work describes and codifies a unifying means of understanding health status. The 2001 version for adults was followed in 2007 by an ICF for children and youth.[4] The ICF is a framework that captures the breadth of issues created by CP and the many arenas of impact.[5] In brief, the ICF considers that each person's function, disability, and health are interdependent and are modified by both environmental and personal factors. Thus, the ICF provides descriptions in 3 major domains of body function, body structure, and activities and participation (execution of tasks and activities and involvement in a life situation). These domains are further clarified with contextual factors, either personal or environmental. ICF domains have been used to understand

and describe the many impacts of CP for individuals and allow for categorization of various CP outcome measures by the domain that is being assessed.

Use of the ICF in CP outcome measurement might best be understood with an example. Consider the use of botulinum toxin in a child with spastic diparetic CP and an abnormal gait. A range of concepts across the ICF spectrum might be altered by use of botulinum toxin and each of these concepts could be assessed using different outcome measures or assessment tools (**Table 1**). This example demonstrates the utility of the ICF in capturing the range of issues for children with CP.

The attention to these concepts has resulted in greater understanding of the relationships between the domains of the ICF in CP. Notably, work has demonstrated that a there is no fixed relationship between the domains of the ICF. Although improvement at the level of body function or activity may take place (for example, decreased spasticity and better gross motor function), this does not necessarily mean improved participation or family satisfaction.[8,9] Furthermore, severity of impairment or disability is not correlated directly with quality of life.[10] These findings might seem surprising when viewed through the lens of a purely medical model, but in the light of the ICF, a far more nuanced understanding of the interplay of these factors is possible.

Selecting Measures

Variety

Choosing the most appropriate outcome measures or assessment tools in clinical research or the clinical care of CP is challenging. With a vast array of areas of interest, many tools have been developed and are being used. Many outcome measures in current use are fairly specific for 1 domain of the ICF, whereas others may span 2 or more domains. Some measures have been carefully designed, validated, and found reliable whereas others were developed casually and have not been rigorously evaluated for their performance. Some measures require special equipment, trained assessors, or lengthy periods of administration; these measures may be less attractive to use due to the costs or inconveniences associated with them. Clinicians and researchers alike must think critically about the available tests, studies, questionnaires, evaluations, interviews, and technologies, and they must consider the patient or subject, the situation, and the question at hand before making selections.

Table 1
International classification of functioning, disability and health domains and outcomes in an example of botulinum toxin treatment in spastic diparetic cerebral palsy

Domain	Possible Effects of Botulinum Toxin	Assessment of Effect
Body structure	Altered muscle structure Cortical reorganization	Muscle biopsy fMRI
Body function	Spasticity reduction Weakness	Tardieu or Ashworth scales Dynamometry
Activity	Change in ambulation Improved gross motor skills	Various gait scales GMFM[6]
Participation	Playing on a soccer team Attending social events	Children's Assessment of Participation and Enjoyment[7]
Environmental contextual factors[a]	Accessible school buildings Transportation to therapy	Questionnaires or review of public policy

[a] Unlikely to change with botulinum toxin injection but included as an illustration.

Quality

When considering outcome measures, it is necessary to evaluate the psychometric performance of each measure. The best measure is one that addresses the domain of concern, is valid and reliable, can be used readily, and is responsive to change. For many measures, some of these criteria are not yet fulfilled. Validity and reliability are key concepts in outcome measurement that demonstrate the measure is truly assessing the concepts of interest and that the assessments are accurate and repeatable. Many measures have been evaluated for validity and reliability in at least a preliminary fashion. Even so, caution must be paid to using each instrument in the manner it was intended, which means administering each measure precisely as the developers instruct and as it was used in the validation studies, including avoiding the use of tool subscales if the subscales have not been demonstrated to stand alone, using the measure in intended populations, and administering the measure as recommended. Some measures are best described as classifications. For example, the Gross Motor Function Classification System (GMFCS) delineates 5 strata of motor functioning in children and youth with CP.[11] It is convenient and widely used to describe severity of impairment in CP, but it has not demonstrated utility nor was it designed to detect changes over time or after interventions. The ability to pick up differences over time is called responsiveness or sensitivity to change. This concept is not well studied in most CP outcome measures.

Application

An additional concern in outcome measures and CP research is the need to match the right measure to an appropriate study design. The desire for greater information about clinical prognosis, natural history, and effects of intervention is sizable and many researchers strive to provide answers. Unfortunately, if studies are not designed well, much effort and many resources may be expended without yielding useful evidence to propel knowledge. In CP research, many studies lack basic design elements, such as defining a primary outcome measure (the main thing that the study intends to evaluate for change) or power calculations (to assure that the study has the right number of subjects to answer the research question efficiently). Many studies do not create high-level evidence because they do not use high-quality design features, including randomization, blinding, allocation concealment, prospective recruitment, and adequate follow-up periods. Thus, without care in study design, the selection of the perfect outcome measure does not assure that a study is of value. Of late, there has been an emphasis also on studying CP interventions using pragmatic trials as part of comparative effectiveness research (CER), which looks at patient preferences when offered typical treatments for a practical clinical scenario.

EXAMPLES OF COMMON OUTCOME MEASURES USED IN CEREBRAL PALSY CLINICAL CARE AND RESEARCH

Dozens of measures are used in the care and research of childhood CP. The items discussed are some of the more common outcome measures and are provided as examples. This list is no way exhaustive nor should it be interpreted as a compendium of the most effective or popular measures. A primary tenet of this article is the concept that outcome measurement in CP is complex and decisions about which assessments should be used must be informed by the patient or subject population and the goals of the evaluation. Measures are reviewed based on the primary ICF domain they address.

Body Structure

Body structure is not commonly evaluated in CP clinical trials. Although most children have brain imaging to support their diagnoses of CP, subsequent evaluations are infrequent. In some settings, particularly for research, functional magnetic resonance imaging (fMRI), diffusion tensor imaging, transcranial magnetic stimulation, magneto-encephalography, and other measures of brain physiology and activity are used.[12,13] Understanding how these measures relate to other outcomes or how to apply them clinically is growing rapidly. Other body structure measures could include biopsy of tissue for chemical or other analyses, radiographic imaging to quantify skeletal deformity, assessments of bone mineral density, or many others.

Body Function

Body function is a frequent arena for CP outcome measures. Spasticity treatments are common in CP care, and various means of evaluation include the Ashworth Scale and Tardieu Scale. These scales are determined by physically moving joints and describing the ease and range of movement. The Ashworth Scale and Modified Ashworth Scale have limited reliability, and their validity is largely unproved (in part because spasticity has long been challenging to quantify).[14] The Tardieu scale may be somewhat less unreliable.[15] Despite the obvious shortcomings of these spasticity measures, they are almost universally used in clinical and research settings for CP. This state of affairs is due to the lack of better performing assessments of spasticity that are easy to use. Strength often is measured using dynamometry. Various dynamometers and techniques are available to directly measure force generation, and some are easier to use or are more reliable than others. The true utility of dynamometry for use in CP is promising but not well established.[16] Strength measurement is used variably in therapy settings and for some research. Range of motion may be assessed with goniometry, using a handheld device held alongside a child's limb to measure angles. Goniometry varies in reliability in research settings for children with CP,[17,18] although it continues to be used in clinical settings.

Activity

Activity measures are used less frequently in clinical settings, probably due to the time and training required for administration, but are ubiquitous in clinical effectiveness studies. The Gross Motor Function Measure (GMFM)[6] is a therapist-administered battery of physical tasks that has established reliability and validity.[19] It takes up to an hour to complete (less in some formats[20]) but provides interval data quantifying a child's status that can be compared with motor development curves for CP.[21] The Pediatric Evaluation of Disability Inventory is a structured interview that generates scores in arenas of self-care, mobility, and social functioning,[22] with evidence of reliability, validity, and responsiveness.

Participation

The Canadian Occupational Performance Measure may be assigned to the activity or participation domains. It assesses individuals' perspectives on tasks of daily life and leisure as well as the individuals' satisfaction with their performance.[23] This measure is unique because it creates individualized priorities rather than evaluating the same tasks or actions for each participant. Reliability, validity, and responsiveness are established.

Most participation measures[24] in use for children have adequate reliability and validity,[25] with less demonstrated responsiveness. The Children's Assessment of

Participation and Enjoyment examines which activities and interests children are pursuing as well as children's enjoyment of the things they do.[7] This survey catalogs information approximately 55 activities, including what, where, when, and how often, in order to describe participation.

Health Status

General health or health status measures include several questionnaires. Some are generic measures that are broadly applied to pediatric populations. These include the Pediatric Quality of Life Inventory,[26] a questionnaire with physical and psychosocial subscales that may be completed by the child or a parent proxy. Another generic measure is the KIDSCREEN, which addresses health-related quality of life with a questionnaire, again available for children or parents.[27] Among the disease-specific health status measures are the Cerebral Palsy Quality of Life Questionnaire for Children (CP-QOL)[28] and the Caregiver Priorities and Child Health Index of Life with Disabilities (CP-CHILD).[29] The CP-QOL is a questionnaire, for parent or child completion, directed at quality of life in general rather than the more specific concept of health-related quality of life. The CP-CHILD measures health status and burden of care for children with severe impairments and is completed by a parent. Each of these questionnaires has been evaluated for validity and reliability.

Core Sets of Measures

In an effort to provide a comprehensive understanding of medical, functional, and health status in CP, researchers have pursued sets of measures that complement each another and reflect a broad range of constructs. Some research has utilized the ICF to organize measures and suggested a tool box of 25 of the most useful measures.[30] More recently, through a collaboration of governmental and professional organizations, a specific set of common data elements was published with the specific intent of use in clinical research.[31]

Classification

Lastly, classification measures have become common mechanisms for describing children with CP.[32] In lieu of or in addition to anatomic descriptions of CP, such as spastic diplegia or dystonic quadriparesis, researchers and clinicians have adopted function-based classifications. The most common schema is the GMFCS.[33] The GMFCS is reliable, stable, and easy to use, such that parents can accurately classify children with CP into the 5 strata of functioning. The highest functioning stratum, I, includes children who walk without restrictions but have limitations in advanced motor skills. The lowest stratum is V and includes children who have severely limited self-mobility, even with assistive technology. Similar classification systems have been developed for manual abilities,[34] communication,[35] and eating and drinking.[36]

UNDERSTANDING CHANGE IN CEREBRAL PALSY

Beyond simply describing an individual's status, the evaluation of change is the primary reason to use outcome measurement. Clinicians, researchers, and especially children and parents want to know if something is different with the passing of time or after a treatment. In CP, understanding change is a complex endeavor. Interventions for CP are not curative, at least with current medical science. This means that change must be looked for in the symptoms or impacts of CP, but dramatic resolution of CP or its associated disability cannot be expected. Assessing change in CP is more subtle than change in some other diagnoses, such as resolving high blood pressure after taking medication. As discussed previously, most individuals with CP have multiple domains of concern that range across the ICF.

Growth and Development as Confounders

Even within any given domain, assessing change requires careful study. Children with CP are truly moving targets. Their function and well-being are expected to change as they grow, develop, and mature. Some of these changes are the result of typical development and may mirror typically developing children or at least resemble typical development. Other changes are a direct consequence of the impairments of CP and reflect significant delay or deviance from typical development. These changes often are described as the natural history of CP. Because children with CP are expected to change, any change that is established over time may simply be the result of natural maturation or development. The pace and degree of change are generally not well understood such that highly reliable predictions can be made. Without this ability to prognosticate accurately, clinicians and researchers cannot establish if changes that follow a treatment of CP are the result of the treatment or would have occurred despite the treatment and are just natural history. The GMFM has been analyzed to produce CP-specific motor development curves that demonstrate the pace and extent of gross motor skill acquisition throughout childhood.[21] This is notable because it is a rare CP measure that has established predictable behavior over time such that a change from expected can be determined. When working with populations of children with CP, studies that use randomized designs control for natural history changes over time, but otherwise it is challenging to differentiate the effects of interventions from the direct effects of CP and development.

Clinical Significance

Another tension in defining change in CP is the issue of significance. Research may be conducted to evaluate an intervention and the results may indicate a statistical effect. This statistical effect would reflect a mathematical likelihood that change occurred with the intervention in terms of the outcome measurements. This mathematical happenstance, however, may or may not reflect a sufficient clinical change to justify the intervention. This concern is not frequent in CP research due to small sample sizes in most studies, but it remains salient. Consider a study that demonstrated a statistically significant improvement in knee-knee distance after botulinum toxin injection to the hip adductors.[37] The increase in knee separation was statistically analyzed and had changed from before to after, with an average increase of 10 cm. Some people argue that increasing separation between knees by such a distance is not enough to make positioning, dressing, or diaper changes truly better. This could be an example of a finding that is statistically significant but not clinically significant. Ultimately, what is of interest also is whether the amount of change is meaningful to the patient and caregiver/family member.

Responsiveness

When measuring change, some sort of ruler must be used. In CP research, many different outcome measures are used in this capacity. Most instruments have been evaluated to confirm that they truly measure what they are intended to measure and have established validity. Many of them, however, have not been evaluated for responsiveness. In an ideal setting, an outcome measure would be used in a population of subjects who are expected to show change to varying degrees. Additional means of evaluating change, maybe even a gold standard, would be used concurrently with the outcome measure and the data from each type of assessment compared. If the outcome measure scores changed in similar ways and with similar scope to the other assessments, then the outcome measure could be declared sensitive to change. Most measures used in CP have not been evaluated in this fashion. Thus, the numbers of outcome measures that have clearly demonstrated adequate responsiveness are low.

Meaningful Change

Tied to the idea of responsiveness is the concept of minimal clinically important differences. These differences are the amount a score on a measure needs to increase or decrease in order to reflect a change in status that is appreciable at a clinical level.[38] Very, very few of the instruments in wide use for CP have been studied to establish a minimal clinically important difference.[39] The best way to define these differences is to follow individuals with repeated evaluations both with the measure that is being studied and with some other means of establishing if an individual has changed in a meaningful manner. Outcome measure scores from the subjects who experience minimal clinical changes then are used to calculate the minimal clinically important difference. When this calculation has been made and a meaningful change score is defined, it is easier to design studies in terms of selecting sample sizes because the power calculations are straightforward. Moreover, clinical care is better informed when change scores can be compared with established minimal clinically important differences.

SUMMARY

Outcome measurement may be the greatest hurdle in research and clinical management of CP. Fortunately, the number and quality of measures continue to increase. With attention to the vast number of impacts of CP, the variability of CP manifestations, and the needs for valid, reliable, and responsive means of measuring the status of children with CP, more valuable outcome measures emerge. The wise application of available outcome measures in optimized settings and thoughtful studies will lead to greater understanding of children with CP and the best management of their disabilities.

DISCLOSURE STATEMENT

The author has nothing to disclose.

REFERENCES

1. Colver A, Rapp M, Eisemann N, et al. Self-reported quality of life of adolescents with cerebral palsy: a cross-sectional and longitudinal analysis. Lancet 2015;385: 705–16.
2. Raina P, O'Donnell M, Rosenbaum P, et al. The health and well-being of caregivers of children with cerebral palsy. Pediatrics 2005;115:e626.
3. World Health Organization. The international classification of functioning, disability and health (ICF). Geneva (Switzerland): World Health Organization; 2001.
4. World Health Organization. International classification of functioning, disability and health - children & youth version (ICF-CY). Geneva (Switzerland): World Health Organization; 2007.
5. Vargus-Adams J, Majnemer A. International Classification of Functioning, Disability and Health (ICF) as a framework for change: revolutionizing rehabilitation. J Child Neurol 2014;29:1030–5.

6. Russell DJ, Rosenbaum PL, Avery LM, et al. Gross Motor function measure (GMFM-66 and GMFM-88) user's manual. In: Clinics in developmental medicine, vol. 159. London: MacKeith Press; 2002.

7. King GA, Law M, King S, et al. Measuring children's participation in recreation and leisure activities: construct validation of the CAPE and PAC. Child Care Health Dev 2007;33:28.

8. Bjornson K, Hays R, Graubert C, et al. Botulinum toxin for spasticity in children with cerebral palsy: a comprehensive evaluation. Pediatrics 2007;120:49.

9. Wright V, Rosenbaum P. How do changes in body functions and structures, activity, and participation relate in children with cerebral palsy. Dev Med Child Neurol 2008;50:283–9.

10. Rapp M, Eisemann N, Arnaud C, et al. Predictors of parent-reported quality of life of adolescents with cerebral palsy: a longitudinal study. Res Dev Disabil 2017;62: 259–70.

11. Palisano R, Rosenbaum P, Walter S, et al. Development and reliability of a system to classify gross motor function in children with cerebral palsy. Dev Med Child Neurol 1997;39:214.

12. Smyser CD, Wheelock MD, Limbrick DD, et al. Neonatal brain injury and aberrant connectivity. Neuroimage 2019;185:609–23.

13. Dubois J, Adibpour P, Poupon C, et al. MRI and M/EEG studies of the white matter development in human fetuses and infants: review and opinion. Brain Plast 2016;2:49–69.

14. Clopton N, Dutton J, Featherston T, et al. Interrater and intrarater reliability of the Modified Ashworth Scale in children with hypertonia. Pediatr Phys Ther 2005; 17:268.

15. Haugh AB, Pandyan AD, Johnson GR. A systematic review of the Tardieu Scale for the measurement of spasticity. Disabil Rehabil 2006;28:899.

16. Mulder-Brouwer AN, Rameckers EA, Bastiaenen CH. Lower extremity handheld dynamometry strength measurement in children with cerebral palsy. Pediatr Phys Ther 2016;28:136–53.

17. Glanzman AM, Swenson AE, Kim H. Intrarater range of motion reliability in cerebral palsy: a comparison of assessment methods. Pediatr Phys Ther 2008; 20:369.

18. Ten Berge SR, Halbertsma JP, Maathuis PG, et al. Reliability of popliteal angle measurement: a study in cerebral palsy patients and healthy controls. J Pediatr Orthop 2007;27:648.

19. Russell DJ, Avery LM, Rosenbaum PL, et al. Improved scaling of the gross motor function measure for children with cerebral palsy: evidence of reliability and validity. Phys Ther 2000;80:873.

20. Avery LM, Russell DJ, Rosenbaum PL. Criterion validity of the GMFM-66 item set and the GMFM-66 basal and ceiling approaches for estimating GMFM-66 scores. Dev Med Child Neurol 2013;55:534–8.

21. Rosenbaum PL, Walter SD, Hanna SE, et al. Prognosis for gross motor function in cerebral palsy: creation of motor development curves. JAMA 2002;288:1357.

22. Haley S, Coster W, Ludlow L. Pediatric evaluation of disability inventory (PEDI), Version 1: development, standardization and administration manual. Boston: New England Medical Center, PEDI Research Group; 1992.

23. Law M, Baptiste S, McColl M, et al. The Canadian occupational performance measure: an outcome measure for occupational therapy. Can J Occup Ther 1990; 57:82.

24. Chien CW, Rodger S, Copley J, et al. Comparative content review of children's participation measures using the international classification of functioning, disability and health - children and youth. Arch Phys Med Rehabil 2014;95:141–52.

25. Sakzewski L, Boyd R, Ziviani J. Clinimetric properties of participation measures for 5- to 13-year-old children with cerebral palsy: a systematic review. Dev Med Child Neurol 2007;49:232.

26. Varni JW, Seid M, Kurtin PS. PedsQL 4.0: reliability and validity of the Pediatric Quality of Life Inventory version 4.0 generic core scales in healthy and patient populations. Med Care 2001;39:800.

27. Robitail S, Simeoni MC, Erhart M, et al. Validation of the European proxy KIDSCREEN-52 pilot test health-related quality of life questionnaire: first results. J Adolesc Health 2006;39:596.e1.

28. Waters E, Davis E, Reddihough D, et al. A new condition specific quality of life scale for children with cerebral palsy. Patient Reported Outcomes Newsletter 2005;35:10.

29. Narayanan UG, Fehlings D, Weir S, et al. Initial development and validation of the Caregiver Priorities and Child Health Index of Life with Disabilities (CPCHILD). Dev Med Child Neurol 2006;48:804.

30. Schiariti V, Tatla S, Sauve K, et al. Toolbox of multiple-item measures aligning with the ICF Core Sets for children and youth with cerebral palsy. Eur J Paediatr Neurol 2017;21:252–63.

31. Schiariti V, Fowler E, Brandenberg JE, et al. A common data language for clinical research studies: the National Institute of Neurological Disorders and Stroke and American Academy for Cerebral Palsy and Developmental Medicine Cerebral Palsy Common Data Elements Version 1.0 recommendations. Dev Med Child Neurol 2018;60:976–86.

32. Paulson A, Vargus-Adams J. Overview of four functional classification systems commonly used in cerebral palsy. Children 2017;4:30.

33. Palisano R, Cameron D, Rosenbaum P, et al. Stability of the gross motor function classification system [abstract]. Dev Med Child Neurol 2004;46(Suppl 99):4.

34. Eliasson AC, Krumlinde-Sundholm L, Rosblad B, et al. The Manual Ability Classification System (MACS) for children with cerebral palsy: scale development and evidence of validity and reliability. Dev Med Child Neurol 2006;48:549.

35. Hidecker MJC, Paneth N, Rosenbaum P, et al. Developing a classification tool of functional communication in individuals with cerebral palsy. Dev Med Child Neurol 2008;50:43.

36. Sellers D, Mandy A, Pennington L, et al. Development and reliability of a system to classify the eating and drinking ability of people with cerebral palsy. Dev Med Child Neurol 2014;56:245–51.

37. Mall V, Heinen F, Siebel A, et al. Treatment of adductor spasticity with BTX-A in children with CP: a randomized, double-blind, placebo-controlled study. Dev Med Child Neurol 2006;48:10.

38. Beaton DE, Bombardier C, Katz JN, et al. Looking for important change/differences in studies of responsiveness. OMERACT MCID Working Group. Outcome Measures in Rheumatology. Minimal Clinically Important Difference. J Rheumatol 2001;28:400.

39. Oeffinger D, Bagley A, Rogers S, et al. Outcome tools used for ambulatory children with cerebral palsy: responsiveness and minimum clinically important differences. Dev Med Child Neurol 2008;50:918–25.

Adaptive Sports, Arts, Recreation, and Community Engagement

Stephanie Tow, MD[a],*, Joslyn Gober, DO[b], Maureen R. Nelson, MD[c]

KEYWORDS

- Adaptive performance • Adaptive recreation • Adaptive sports
- Adaptive sports medicine • Cerebral palsy

KEY POINTS

- This article discusses the history of adaptive sports and recreational activities.
- This article reviews the importance, physiologic impacts, and psychosocial benefits of adaptive sports and recreational activities for individuals with cerebral palsy.
- This article reviews the barriers and medical challenges faced by individuals with cerebral palsy in regards to exercise, adaptive sports, and recreation.
- This article discusses the various activities available for individuals with cerebral palsy, including camps, sports, arts, and parks.
- This article provides a list of available resources for adaptive sports and recreational opportunities.

 Video content accompanies this article at http://www.pmr.theclinics.com.

INTRODUCTION

Sports and recreational activities play a vital role for all individuals, and those with cerebral palsy (CP) are no different. Although those with CP may face barriers to participation and be at risk for injuries or complications, it is suggested that involvement in these activities are beneficial. Providing both physiologic and psychosocial benefits,

Drs J. Gober and S. Tow contributed equally to the article and are joint primary authors.
Disclosure Statement: The authors have nothing to disclose.
[a] Sports Medicine Center, Department of Orthopedics, Children's Mercy Kansas City, 2401 Gillham Road, Kansas City, MO 64108, USA; [b] Department of Physical Medicine and Rehabilitation, Baylor College of Medicine, Texas Children's Hospital, 6701 Fannin Street, Suite 1280, Houston, TX 77030, USA; [c] Department of Physical Medicine and Rehabilitation, Baylor College of Medicine, Children's Hospital of San Antonio, 315 North San Saba, Suite 1135, San Antonio, TX 78207, USA
* Corresponding author.
E-mail address: stephanie.tow@gmail.com

Phys Med Rehabil Clin N Am 31 (2020) 143–158
https://doi.org/10.1016/j.pmr.2019.09.003
1047-9651/20/© 2019 Elsevier Inc. All rights reserved.

adaptive sports and recreational activities are important in providing the best quality of life.

HISTORY

Adaptive sports and athletics began in the nineteenth century and have developed significantly throughout the years.Kaitz and Miller detail the historical progression well throughout their chapter of "Adaptive Sports and Recreation" in Pediatric Rehabilitation[1]: In 1888, the Sports Club for the Deaf was established in Berlin, Germany as the first adaptive organization, and the first international competition, known as the International Silent Games, was created in 1924. Gradually, more associations were established. In 1940, wheelchair polo was invented in England, leading quickly to the development of wheelchair basketball. War veterans in the Unites States began playing basketball around that same time, which soon resulted in the establishment of the National Wheelchair Athletic Association, now called "Adaptive Sports USA."

In 1948, Dr Tim Nugent pioneered programs for World War II veterans with physical disabilities, which quickly opened to nonveterans. These programs included wheelchair sports for bowling, baseball, football, and basketball. Dr Nugent began the first men's collegiate wheelchair basketball team, and the first National Wheelchair Basketball tournament was held the following year. Instituting wheelchair athletics initiated the development of the first accessible dormitories, accessible bus systems, and universal accessibility standards. In 1948, the first international sporting event for athletes of various disabilities was established: the Stoke Mandeville Games for the paralyzed, in which 16 athletes competed in wheelchair basketball, archery, and table tennis. In 1960, the United States made their international debut at the first Paralympic Games in Rome.

As the years have passed, the amount of adaptive sport and recreational activities has grown. In 1967, the National Handicapped Sports and Recreation Association was formed to address the needs of winter athletes, and it has since been reorganized as "Disabled Sports USA." The Amateur Sports Act, or Public Law 95-606, was passed in 1978, recognizing athletes with disabilities as part of the Olympic movement.

The United States Cerebral Palsy Athletic Association was developed in the 1970s. In the 1980s, the National Wheelchair Athletic Association created a junior division to include ages 6 to 18. Since then, junior level participation and programming have been implemented into other organizations. There are increasingly available activities in the community through the Adapted Physical Educations (APE) program. APE was developed in response to the Individuals with Disabilities Education Act, stating that children with disabilities have the right to "free, appropriate public education in the least restrictive environment."[1] It passed in 1990, mandating that children with disabilities have the same opportunity for education as others, including physical activities.

IMPORTANCE/BENEFITS

Individuals with CP have varying degrees of motor and sensory deficits, epilepsy, intellectual impairments, learning and attention difficulties, and musculoskeletal abnormalities.[2] These deficits result in limitations of motor control, balance, posture, strength, and endurance, which may reduce participation in physical and social activities, leading to a more sedentary lifestyle, and increase the risk of obesity. People with CP who lack opportunities to incorporate healthy, exercise-based movement patterns are at higher risk for fatigue, injury, or pain secondary to maladaptation to their most impaired body parts.[3] In particular, individuals with CP are at risk for postimpairment syndrome, a combination of fatigue, muscle weakness, and pain associated with congenital brain injury, which when combined with decreased physical activity, may lead to maladaptation to their most impaired side or body parts.[4] It is, therefore, important to introduce healthy exercise habits to individuals with CP early to counter these risks associated with physical inactivity.

Physiologic Impact

In children without disabilities, exercise demonstrated significant improvements in aerobic endurance, static strength, flexibility, and equilibrium.[1] Historically, it was thought that children with CP were negatively impacted by strengthening exercises, exacerbating weakness and spasticity. However, recent studies have shown beneficial effects. For example, ambulatory patients with CP who participate in circuit training show improved aerobic and anaerobic capacity, muscle strength, health-related quality-of-life scores, body image, and walking efficiency.[5–8] Continued long-term exercise participation may also help individuals with CP maintain their optimal neuromuscular function throughout life.[9] Moreover, it has been demonstrated that individuals with disabilities who participate in sports have improved strength, stamina,[10–12] cardiovascular health, fitness,[10,13,14] and decreased secondary health conditions.[10,14,15]

Psychosocial Impact

Many studies have demonstrated increased social isolation with fewer friendships among those with disabilities.[1] Adaptive sports and recreation provide beneficial psychosocial impacts for these children. It may improve psychological well-being, mood and emotions, peer and social support, while also decreasing experiences of being bullied.[16] Athletes with impairments have also been shown to have increased psychological resilience, finding ways to successfully navigate life tasks in the face of social disadvantage or other adverse conditions. For instance, athletes with disabilities may have decreased physiologic responses to pain compared with athletes without disabilities because of their increased resilience serving as a protective factor in response to pain or acute injury.[2] Increased psychological resilience may be especially helpful for those who have chronic pain, but should also be cautioned because medical attention may not be sought for more severe injuries due to their decreased perception of pain.

BARRIERS

In children with disabilities, the amount of physical activity is restricted by the underlying disability, physical barriers, and availability.[17] The most commonly cited barriers are lack of local facilities, limited physical access and appropriate equipment, attitudinal barriers by public and staff, lack of trained personnel or programs with adequate supervision, and financial concerns.[18] Other barriers include impaired awareness of resources, parental concerns, personal motivation, and underestimating one's ability to be able to participate in adaptive activities.

MEDICAL CHALLENGES

In general, athletes with CP face more medical challenges than athletes without disabilities. Each athlete with CP may be at risk for different medical issues and injuries, depending on the clinical presentation of their CP, their comorbidities, and their sport. Seizures, intellectual impairment, impaired walking ability, and communication difficulties predict lower levels of physical activity among children with CP.[19]

Musculoskeletal Issues

Individuals with CP often have abnormal tone, decreased joint range of motion or contractures, decreased neuromuscular control of movement, impaired coordination, and muscle weakness, all of which contribute to risk for musculoskeletal injury and impaired exercise performance. Athletes with CP have a higher risk of musculoskeletal injury in both the upper and the lower limbs, with hypertonia often being the causative factor.[4] Abnormal muscle tone and decreased range of motion in CP lead to abnormal loads on joints, causing pain and injuries.[20–22] Patellofemoral pain syndrome is commonly experienced by older athletes with CP because of spasticity of the quadriceps causing an abnormally high load on the patella, leading to patella maltracking in the trochlear groove and resulting in damage of the retropatellar cartilage.[23] Injuries and pain also result from other muscles with normal tone compensating for these muscles with abnormal tone.

Athletes with CP not only face abnormal biomechanical stresses from abnormal muscle tone but also may have abnormal joint positioning that predisposes them to injuries. For example, individuals with CP commonly have ankle and foot deformities, which increase the risk of ankle instability, metatarsalgia, and an increase in overload areas of the foot complex.[24]

In the Paralympic Games in London 2012, Sochi 2014, and Rio 2016, seated para-athletes tended to have upper-limb injuries, whereas ambulatory para-athletes tended to have lower-limb injuries.[25] Men and women had similar overall injury rates.[26] The most common injuries were sprains, strains, blisters, and lacerations.[26] In track and field events in paraathletics, ambulant athletes with CP had a lower overall injury incidence rate compared with ambulant athletes in other impairment categories.[26]

Early onset osteoarthritis is another common musculoskeletal issue those with CP face.[27] With abnormal muscle tone, less muscle activation, and muscle weakness, joints experience a decrease in the protective action of the surrounding musculature, thereby increasing the risk of injury and degeneration of these joints.[28] The joints most commonly affected include the low back, hip, knee, and ankle/foot complex.[20] Athletic training at the elite level may further increase the risk of osteoarthritis with high mechanical loads placed on joints during extensive training and competition.[29] Compensatory techniques and improper form may also increase the risk of osteoarthritis on areas of the body not directly affected by CP.

Preventing Musculoskeletal Injuries

There is evidence that long-term exercise participation leads to maintenance of optimal neuromuscular function over an individual's lifespan,[9] which in turn, may decrease the risk of musculoskeletal injury. For those with hemiparetic CP, a standard rehabilitative approach is to rehabilitate and perform exercises on both sides of the individual, at the pace and intensity of the hemiparetic side.[30] This training technique may help avoid compensatory muscle activation of the unaffected side, decreasing risk of injury and early onset osteoarthritis of this side. For all types of CP, special attention should be made to appropriately stretch as taught by a physical therapist.[31] For most individuals with CP, flexion patterns often dominate, and so strength training should also be focused on extension exercise.[31] Most research on injury patterns in adaptive sports has been conducted at the elite level, which is helpful when considering injury prevention programs for these athletes.[20] However, further research is needed for adaptive athletes at youth, recreational, and less competitive levels to better serve and support these athletes.

Pain

Pain is frequently reported in individuals with CP and interferes with participation in both activities of daily living and physical activity.[31] The most common areas of pain are the lower limb, hip, and low back and are thought to be related to abnormal tone associated with CP.[32,33] Athletes with CP who have chronic pain should work with their physician to develop a treatment plan for the underlying cause of pain and/or a comprehensive pain management plan that may incorporate an appropriate exercise routine. There is a wide range of treatment options for pain in CP, depending on the cause and severity of pain. These treatment options include but are not limited to ice, stretching, physical therapy, transcutaneous electrical nerve stimulation, oral pain medications ranging from acetaminophen and nonsteroidal anti-inflammatory drugs to opiates, oral spasticity/dystonia medications, chemodenervation, spinal cord stimulators, implantable pumps for either intrathecal morphine and/or baclofen, orthopedic surgery, and selective dorsal rhizotomy.

Fatigue and Maximal Exertion

Athletes with CP also commonly report fatigue, which may have both physiologic and pathologic components.[34] As athletes fatigue, posture and form may be compromised, which may increase the risk of injury. In addition, acute spasmodic reaction following an intense competition has also been seen in athletes with CP,[20] usually toward the end of an event. This acute spasmodic reaction also may be secondary to muscle fatigue and altered biomechanical stressors, leading to further injury.

Other Medical Comorbidities and Illness

To date, most medical illness that has been studied in athletes with disabilities has been at the elite level.[20] When evaluating the percentage of all athletes with illness (incidence proportion of illness) at the Olympic Games versus the Paralympic Games at London 2012, Sochi 2014, and Rio 2016, the incidence proportion of illness is almost twice as high in Paralympic athletes compared with Olympic athletes.[31] Incidence of illness was noted to be significantly higher for Paralympic athletes in the Winter Games (Sochi 2014) compared with the Summer Games (London 2012, Rio 2016).[31] Respiratory illness was the most common medical issue, followed by dermatologic, gastrointestinal, and genitourinary illness.[31] In the Summer Games, the most common organ systems involved in medical illness in Paralympic athletes were the skin, nervous system, and ears/nose/throat.[31] Studies have shown that gender and precompetition versus competition season are not risks for increased illness.[31] Further studies are needed to evaluate the risk of sport code, type of impairment, travel, training load, competition load, nutrition, and personal habits on medical illness.

For athletes with convulsive disorders, particular attention needs to be made in order to avoid dehydration, electrolyte imbalances, emotional stress, hyperventilation, or hypoglycemia, because these factors may lower the threshold for seizures.[31] However, exercise may also have a protective effect on seizures: aerobic exercises lead to increased lactic acid, thus lowering pH and stabilizing membranes, decreasing the risk of seizures.[31]

Other common medical challenges faced by athletes with CP include impaired oral health (eg, drooling), impaired vision and hearing, higher incidence of chronic diseases (eg, hypertension, genitourinary dysfunction) compared with the general population, and depression.[20] Those who are nonambulatory and dependent on a wheelchair for mobility also have a higher risk of scoliosis, hip dysplasia/subluxation, low back pain, and skin breakdown.[20] Because athletes with CP may also be on multiple medications because of various comorbidities, side effects need to be cautioned more than in the population of athletes without disabilities, who generally have less comorbidities and therefore are not on as many medications, if any.

PHYSIATRISTS' ROLE

Physiatrists have extensive medical expertise in serving individuals with disabilities and their medical needs to help them achieve functional goals and an optimal quality of life in the context of their physical impairments. Pediatric physiatrists, in particular, specialize in the care of children and sometimes adults who have developmental disabilities. With comprehensive musculoskeletal training, physiatrists are also able to care for the exercise and athletic needs of those with and without disabilities. Given the aforementioned medical issues, which may sometimes be complex, and risks for musculoskeletal injury, individuals with CP who are interested in becoming more physically active should be evaluated by a physiatrist to address their needs to prevent injuries and promote their performance.

SPORTS AND EXERCISE

At the national level, there are many adaptive sports opportunities ranging from the beginner/recreational level to the elite/competitive level. US Paralympics[35] offers various summer and winter sports, for which individuals with CP may meet criteria to participate, depending on their impairment. Some sports, such as football 7-a-side and boccia, were designed with athletes with CP in mind, whereas others, such as Paralympic swimming (**Fig. 1**, Video 1), encompass a wide array of diagnoses and impairments. For each sport, there is a classification process to determine (1) eligibility for the sport by the extent of impairment and (2) which class the athlete would

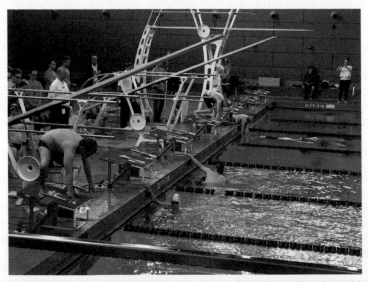

Fig. 1. Paralympic swimmers of a diversity of diagnoses (including CP) with a wide range of impairments taking their mark for a US Paralympic Swimming meet. Start positions for events may vary depending on the swimmer's physical impairment and their classification results.

be classified into for competition. Athletes with CP most commonly fall into one of the impairment categories of hypertonia, ataxia, or athetosis.[34]

Another national resource is the National Sports Center for the Disabled (NSCD),[35] located in Denver, Colorado. This extensive program includes opportunities for adaptive ski (**Fig. 2**, Video 2), water sports, climbing, therapeutic horseback riding, and camps. Individuals with CP involved in this program have a wide range of impairments, and volunteers through the program undergo extensive, rigorous training to best support these individuals while also allowing them as much functional independence as their impairment allows.

There are many local and regional sports programs that include children with CP. Kinetic Kids is 1 such program, located in San Antonio, Texas. Originally founded

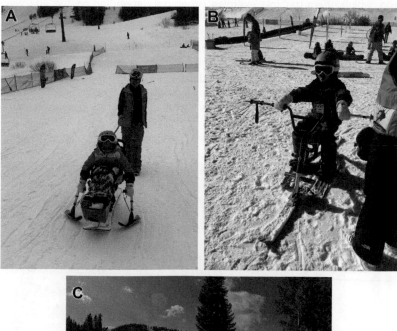

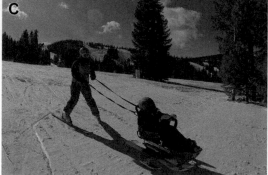

Fig. 2. Various adaptive ski program options are offered through the NSCD at Winter Park, Colorado. (*A*) Adaptive ski volunteer instructor teaching and tethering a sit ski student with CP, teaching her to use her trunk and hand-held outriggers to maneuver a sit ski. The use of hand-held outriggers requires adequate motor control and strength in the upper extremities. (*B*) Adaptive ski student with CP learning how to maneuver a ski bike. (*C*) Adaptive ski volunteer instructor teaching and tethering a sit ski student with CP, teaching her to use her trunk and fixed outriggers to maneuver a sit ski. Fixed outriggers are often used if a student does not have adequate motor control or strength in the upper extremities.

by 2 pediatric physical therapists with just 1 T-ball team of 12 children in 2001, it has since grown to 234 sports and recreation programs (including competitive and recreational opportunities for wheelchair basketball and track, swimming, art, drumming, music, and dance) for more than 2800 children with special needs in 2019 (**Fig. 3**). Their sports and recreation programs are designed to encourage mobility and activity, foster courage and confidence, and boost self-esteem and pride.

To promote exercise and fitness in people with disabilities, more adaptive gyms are developing across the United States. Adaptive gyms are especially needed for the individuals with CP who no longer need physical therapy, but have difficulties performing exercises in a mainstream gym and could benefit from some adaptive equipment and fitness instruction. One example is NeuAbility, an adaptive gym located in Denver, Colorado, which offers multiple exercise programs depending on the adaptive athlete's level of interest.[36]

Technology has also allowed for individuals with CP to perform exercises in the comfort of their homes, using phone apps, social media, or online videos. One example is "Workout Wednesdays with Zach Anner," a comedian with CP who has helped motivate people with and without disabilities around the world to work out.[37] Other examples include the Cerebral Palsy Foundation's Evolve[21] app, which also provides many options for adaptive fitness via its app.[38] For more resources, please see in the below Resources section.

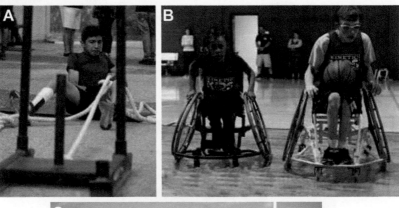

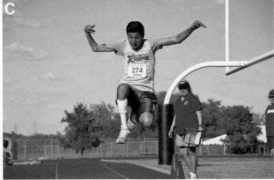

Fig. 3. Kinetic Kids participating in various competitive and recreational activities. (*A*) Cross-fit workout. (*B*) Basketball practice. (*C*) Long jump.

CAMPS

There has been a recent dramatic growth of camps for children and teens with CP, with an increasing breadth of available activities, including fishing, swimming, arts and crafts, drama, dance, academics, photography, sailing, and advanced sports. Information can now be searched by location, activities, ages, and possibility of sibling attendance. Camps vary in the degree of medical support available, from basic to advanced, even supporting those on ventilators. There are also camps for children with CP that incorporate therapeutic methods, such as constraint-induced movement therapy. Some of the camp sources are listed later in the Resources section.

ARTS
Dance

Wheelchair dancing began in 1972, where the wheelchair is considered an extension of the body. Dance has been shown to improve aerobic power, muscle endurance, proprioception, strength, and flexibility; helps with equilibrium and agility as well as gait speed; enhances psychological and emotional states of mind; and improves memory, copying ability, expression, and appreciation.[17,39] Thus, dance not only plays a physical and athletic role but it also acts as a means of artistic expression and can be used as a therapeutic tool, targeting physical, cognitive, and psychological impairments.[40,41]

Movements learned in dance can be transferred to everyday functional mobility. The principles of classical ballet have been used for postural control, trunk stabilization, static and dynamic balance, and focus movement control. It has also been shown to minimize skeletal deformity as well as the loss of endurance, as perceived by parents and therapists.[42,43] In a study investigating the effects of 6 months of dance interventions, results demonstrated that regular participation in dance classes was associated with improvements in posture and reaction times, cognitive and motor performance, as well as subjective well-being.[44]

In addition, dance is inexpensive and does not require any sophisticated equipment.[45] As such, dance should be considered a great activity for children with CP because it has the potential to provide benefits in various aspects of life (**Fig. 4**).

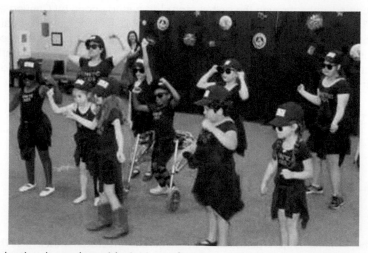

Fig. 4. Adaptive dance class with children of various abilities.

Music

Music is another form of art that plays an important role in social activities, religious ceremonies, or physical expression. Over time, music and instruments have been developed, changed, and advanced, as have music styles. Fortunately, there are many options for adaptations to be made for individuals who want to play music. Adaptations can be as simple as a universal cuff with a holder for drumsticks or as sophisticated as a computer program to put sounds together to form music.[1] A study published in 2003 looked at children with visual impairments who participated in a music program, and it showed an improvement in attention, focus, and arousal.[15]

Theater

Theater is another area to develop social skills as well as physical and cognitive abilities. One program developed for children with special needs is The Penguin Project. It was established in 2004 by Dr Andrew Morgan, a developmental pediatrician and actor, and it has now grown to 27 chapters in 15 states. This program pairs children with special needs with age-level peers in preparing for and performing children's musical theater productions. Children learn songs, dance routines, and dialogue to perform in their shows (**Fig. 5**). Among the goals of the program are to provide an opportunity for children with special needs to develop creative skills related to theater arts, to facilitate interaction between children with special needs and their age level peers, and to provide a form of support and interaction for families of children with special needs. Surveys done with participants and parents have demonstrated that the children felt more proud of themselves, felt more independent, and felt better overall about being different since being a part of this project.[46]

Martial Arts

Martial Arts are movements practiced for a variety of reasons, including self-defense, physical and mental development, or spiritual and cultural connections. It requires complex coordination between different body parts moving in a slow-paced, synchronous, and continuous pattern. These movements can be adapted to suit individuals with physical weakness or disabilities, and they can be modified to allow skills to be trained at the wheelchair level. Children are taught self-respect, self-defense, and control and can advance through the belt system.[1] In a study done by Cheung and colleagues[16] in 2007, individuals with lower-limb disabilities who practiced tai chi for just 4 months resulted in improvement in shoulder range of motion, assumed to be due to increase in strength of muscles and joint flexibility. In addition, martial arts require little space, can be practiced indoors or outdoors, and provide the opportunity for ongoing learning and self-development.

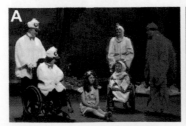
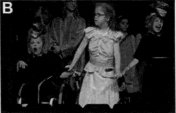

Fig. 5. The Penguin Project performing in numerous theatrical shows. (*A*) The Little Mermaid Jr. (*B*) The Little Mermaid Jr.

PARKS

Morgan's Wonderland describes itself as "the world's first ultra-accessible theme park." Inspired by his daughter, Morgan, Gordon Hartman resolved to create opportunities where those with and without disabilities can come together not only for fun but also for a better understanding of one another. Opening in April 2010, Morgan's Wonderland became the world's first theme park designed with special-needs individuals in mind and built for everyone. It is a completely wheelchair-accessible park featuring more than 25 elements, including rides, playgrounds, and other colorful attractions (**Figs. 6** and **7**). In 2017, Morgan's Inspirational Island was opened as an adjacent water park, and it was named one of the "world's greatest places" by *Time* magazine in 2018.[47] They even offer use of power wheelchairs that can be used in their water park and have trained staff to fit the chairs (**Figs. 8** and **9**).

DEVELOPING/BUILDING NETWORKS

Multiple different models exist in the development of adaptive sports and recreation organizations and how individuals with disabilities access these organizations. Some organizations are based out of hospital systems, while others exist as freestanding nonprofit organizations.

With the assistance of social media, apps, and other technological advances, people and organizations are better able to network across the world to collectively develop adaptive sports organizations or networks. However, although these resources are available to anyone who is motivated to search for them, more encouragement and motivation may be needed for others with disabilities, especially those with a new disability or youth who have not yet been exposed to the adaptive sports and recreation community.

In 2017, a rehabilitation psychologist with a few physiatrists and sports medicine physicians at the University of Texas Southwestern (UTSW) developed its Adaptive Sports Coalition (ASC) in the Dallas/Fort Worth area to better collaborate and network with the wealth of adaptive sports and recreation organizations in the area.[48] Each year, the ASC sponsors a large exposition to showcase the opportunities available through adaptive sports/performance organizations and allows participants to try different adaptive experiences. With UTSW serving as the hub of the ASC, patients with disabilities in their health care system have a more direct connection to these

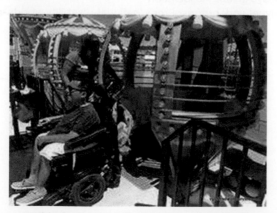

Fig. 6. Enjoying an accessible ferris wheel at Morgan's Wonderland.

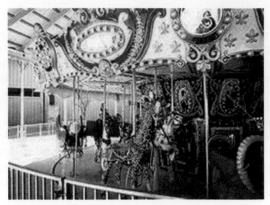

Fig. 7. Accessible merry-go-round at Morgan's Wonderland.

adaptive organizations, providing them with easier access to get involved with these organizations when medically appropriate.

Encouragement of patients to get involved with adaptive sports/recreation/performance opportunities can also be performed in other ways. When appropriate in clinic or hospital settings, clinicians who see patients with disabilities should discuss potential interests in adaptive sports and recreation. By keeping a list of resources for adaptive sports and recreation on hand or accessible in the electronic health record system, clinicians may easily provide helpful resources to individuals with disabilities and make a significant difference in the lifestyle and health of their patients.

USEFUL RESOURCES FOR ADAPTIVE SPORTS AND RECREATION IN CEREBRAL PALSY

Jooay iPhone app
  https://www.child-bright.ca/jooay
American Academy of Physical Medicine & Rehabilitation Directory of Organizations
  for Athletes with Disabilities
  https://www.aapmr.org/about-physiatry/about-physical-medicine-rehabilitation/
    patient-resources/directory-of-organizations-for-athletes-with-disabilites—
    listing
US Cerebral Palsy Athletic Association
  http://cpfamilynetwork.org/resources/national-disability-sports-alliance-ndsa/

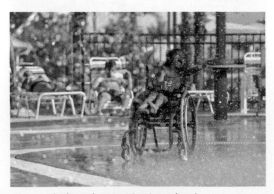

Fig. 8. A child enjoying a splash pad at Inspiration Island.

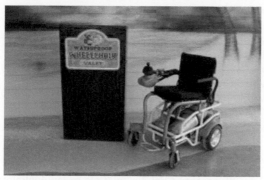

Fig. 9. A pneumatic, waterproof power wheelchair at Inspiration Island.

US Paralympics
   https://www.teamusa.org/us-paralympics.aspx
American Association of Adapted Sports Program (AAASP)
   http://adaptedsports.org/
Disabled Sports USA
   https://www.disabledsportsusa.org/sports/adaptive-sports/
Blaze Sports
   https://www.blazesports.org/
Adaptive Sports USA
   https://adaptivesportsusa.org/
Challenged Athletes Foundation
   https://www.challengedathletes.org/
Winners on Wheels
   http://www.wowusa.com/
Special Olympics
   https://www.specialolympics.org/
Expand Boulder
   https://bouldercolorado.gov/parks-rec/expand-program-for-people-with-disabilities
National Sports Center for the Disabled
   https://nscd.org/
University of Texas Southwestern Adaptive Sports Coalition
   https://www.facebook.com/UTSWAdaptiveSports/
Kinetic Kids
   https://www.kinetickidstx.org/
NeuAbility Adaptive Gym
   https://neuability.org/
Camps for Children with CP
   https://www.veryspecialcamps.com
   https://www.mysummercamps.com/camps/Special_Needs_Camps/Cerebral_
      Palsy/
   https://www.facebook.com/events/TWUSOTADenton/cimt-summer-camp-at-
      scottish-rite/113348999228685/
Workout Wednesdays with Zach Anner
   https://www.youtube.com/watch?v=JqEQ4SSdZAs
Penguin Project
   http://penguinproject.org/
Evolve[21] app by Cerebral Palsy Foundation

https://www.evolve21.org/about-evolve21/
Adaptive Trails
https://adaptivetrails.com/
Adaptive Adventures
https://adaptiveadventures.org/
Wilderness on Wheels
https://www.wildernessonwheels.org/
Cerebral Palsy Foundation Products
https://www.yourcpf.org/all-products/

SUMMARY

Individuals with CP are at increased risk for multiple musculoskeletal and medical issues secondary to their underlying impairments associated with CP. These factors may lead to a more sedentary and isolated lifestyle, increasing the risk of obesity and depression. It is important to incorporate healthy habits, such as routine physical activity, exercise, and involvement in adaptive activities at a young age, to counter these risks. Individuals with CP may face various barriers in accessing adaptive sports and recreation, but with adequate support from the individual's health care providers, resources in the community, and technology, these barriers may be overcome. By understanding the medical challenges individuals with CP encounter, both within and outside of adaptive sports and recreation, ways to better support methods to counter these medical challenges and prevent injury may be found.

SUPPLEMENTARY DATA

Supplementary data related to this article can be found online at https://doi.org/10.1016/j.pmr.2019.09.003.

REFERENCES

1. Kaitz E, Miller M. Adaptive sports and recreation. In: Alexander M, Matthews D, editors. Pediatric rehabilitation. 5th edition. New York: Demos Medical; 2015. p. 79–215.
2. Lopez-Ortiz C, Gaebler-Spira DJ, Mckeeman SN, et al. Dance and rehabilitation in cerebral palsy: a systemic search and review. Dev Med Child Neurol 2019; 61(4):393–8.
3. Runciman P, Tucker R, Ferreira S, et al. Effects of exercise training on performance and function in individuals with cerebral palsy: a critical review. S Afr J Res Sport Ph 2016;38(3):177–93.
4. Runciman P, Tucker R, Ferreira S, et al. The effects of induced volitional fatigue on sprint and jump performance in Paralympic athletes with cerebral palsy. Am J Phys Med Rehabil 2016;95(4):277–90.
5. Verschuren O, Ketelaar M, Gorter JW, et al. Exercise training program in children and adolescents with cerebral palsy: a randomized controlled trial. Arch Pediatr Adolesc Med 2007;161(11):1075–81.
6. Unger M, Faure M, Frieg A. Strength training in adolescent learners with cerebral palsy: a randomized controlled trial. Clin Rehabil 2006;20(6):469–77.
7. Liao HF, Liu YC, Liu WY, et al. Effectiveness of loaded sit-to-stand resistance exercise for children with mild spastic diplegia: a randomized clinical trial. Arch Pediatr Adolesc Med 2007;88(1):25–31.

8. Fowler EG, Kolobe TH, Damiano DL, et al. Promotion of physical fitness and prevention of secondary conditions for children with cerebral palsy: section on pediatric research summit proceedings. Phys Ther 2007;87(11):1495–510.

9. Runciman P, Derman W, Ferreira S, et al. A descriptive comparison of sprint cycling performance and neuromuscular characteristics in able-bodied athletes and paralympic athletes with cerebral palsy. Am J Phys Med Rehabil 2015; 94(1):28–37.

10. Groff DG, Lundberg NR, Zabriskie RB. Influence of adapted sport on quality of life: perceptions of athletes with cerebral palsy. Disabil Rehabil 2009;31(4): 318–26.

11. Taylor NF, Dodd KJ, Larkin H. Adults with cerebral palsy benefit from participating in a strength training programme at a community gymnasium. Disabil Rehabil 2004;26(19):1128–34.

12. Blauwet C, editor. Promoting the health and human rights of individuals with a disability through the Paralympic movement. Bonn (Germany): International Paralympic Committee; 2005.

13. Wells CL, Hooker SP. The spinal injured athlete. Adapt Phys Activ Q 1990;7(3): 249–60.

14. Seaman JA, Corbin C, Pangrazi B. Physical activity and fitness for persons with disabilities, vol. 3. Washington, DC: President's Council on Physical Fitness and Sports Research Digest; 1999. 5.

15. Robb SL. Music interventions and group participation skills of preschoolers with visual impairments: raising questions about music, arousal, and attention. J Music Ther 2003;40(4):266.

16. Cheung SY, Tsai E, Fung L, et al. Physical benefits of Tai Chi Chuan for individuals with lower-limb disabilities. Occup Ther Int 2007;14(1):1–10.

17. Bläsing B, Calvo-Merino B, Cross ES, et al. Neurocognitive control in dance perception and performance. Acta Psychol 2012;139:300–8.

18. Frumberg DB, Gerk AL, Autruong P, et al. Adaptive skiing/snowboarding affects the quality of life of children with disabilities. Palaestra 2019;33(3):21–6.

19. Hammal D, Jarvis SN, Solver AF. Participation of children with cerebral palsy is influences by where they live. Dev Med Child Neurol 2004;46(5):292–8.

20. Graham HK, Rosenbaum P, Paneth N, et al. Cerebral palsy. Nat Rev Dis Primers 2016;2:15082.

21. Sengupta DK, Fan H. The basis of mechanical instability in degenerative disc disease: a cadaveric study of abnormal motion versus load distribution. Spine (Phila Pa 1976) 2014;39(13):1032–43.

22. Ranatunga KW. Skeletal muscle stiffness and contracture in children with spastic cerebral palsy. J Physiol 2011;589(Pt 11):2665.

23. Choi Y, Lee SH, Chung CY, et al. Anterior knee pain in patients with cerebral palsy. Clin Orthop Surg 2014;6(4):426–31.

24. Kedem P, Scher DM. Foot deformities in children with cerebral palsy. Curr Opin Pediatr 2015;27(1):67–74.

25. Tuakli-Wosornu YA, Mashkovskiy E, Ottesen T, et al. Acute and chronic musculoskeletal injury in para sport: a critical review. Tuakli-Wosornu YA, Derman W, eds. Para and Adapted Sports Medicine. Phys Med Rehabil Clin N Am 2018;29(2): 205–43.

26. Blauwet CA, Cushman D, Emery C, et al. Risk of injuries in Paralympic track and field differs by impairment and event discipline: a prospective cohort study at the London 2012 Paralympic Games. Am J Sports Med 2016;44(6):1455–62.

27. Carter DR, Tse B. The pathogenesis of osteoarthritis in cerebral palsy. Dev Med Child Neurol 2009;51(Suppl 4):79–83.
28. Tanaka M, Shigihara Y, Watanabe Y. Central inhibition regulates motor output during physical fatigue. Brain Res 2011;1412:37–43.
29. Gouttebarge V, Inklaar H, Backx F, et al. Prevalence of osteoarthritis in former elite athletes: a systematic overview of the recent literature. Rheumatol Int 2015;35(3):405–18.
30. Brukner P, Khan K. Clinical sports medicine. 3rd edition. Sydney (Australia): McGraw-Hill; 2006.
31. Janse van Rensberg DC, Schwellnus M, Derman W, et al. Illness among paralympic athletes: epidemiology, risk markers, and preventative strategies. Tuakli-Wosornu YA, Derman W, eds. Para and Adapted Sports Medicine. Phys Med Rehabil Clin N Am 2018;29(2):185–203.
32. Brunton LK, Rice CL. Fatigue in cerebral palsy: a critical review. Dev Neurorehabil 2012;15(1):54–62.
33. Jensen MP, Engel JM, Hoffman AJ, et al. Natural history of chronic pain and pain treatment in adults with cerebral palsy. Am J Phys Med Rehabil 2004;83(6):439–45.
34. US Paralympics (2019). Available at: https://www.teamusa.org/US-Paralympics. Accessed January 20, 2019.
35. National Sports Center for the Disabled (2015). Available at: https://nscd.org/about-nscd-adaptive-sports/. Accessed January 20, 2019.
36. NeuAbility (2019). Available at: https://neuability.org/. Accessed January 20, 2019.
37. Anner Z. "Pullups and Pick-me-ups–Workout Wednesday #1" (2013). Available at: https://www.youtube.com/watch?v=JqEQ4SSdZAs. Accessed January 20, 2019.
38. Cerebral Palsy Foundation. Evolve[21] 2019. Available at: https://www.evolve21.org/about-evolve21/. Accessed January 20, 2019.
39. Keogh JW, Kilding A, Pidgeon P, et al. Physical benefits of dancing for healthy older adults: a review. J Aging Phys Act 2009;17:479–500.
40. Ritter M, Low KG. Effects of dance/movement therapy: a metaanalysis. Arts Psychother 1996;23:249–60.
41. Strassel J, Cherkin D, Steuten L, et al. A systematic review of the evidence for the effectiveness of dance therapy. Altern Ther Health Med 2011;17:50–9.
42. Lopez-Ortiz C, Gladden K, Deon L, et al. Dance program for physical rehabilitation and participation in children with cerebral palsy. Arts Health 2012;4:39–54.
43. Lopez-Ortiz C, Egan T, Gaebler–Spira DJ. Pilot study of a targeted dance class for physical rehabilitation in children with cerebral palsy. Sage Open Med 2016;4:1–5.
44. Kattenstroth JC, Kalisch T, Holt S, et al. Six months of dance intervention enhances postural, sensorimotor, and cognitive performance in elderly without affecting cardio-respiratory functions. Front Aging Neurosci 2013;5:5.
45. Demers M, Thomas A, Wittich W, et al. Implementing a novel dance intervention in rehabilitation: perceived barriers and facilitators. Disabil Rehabil 2015;37(12):1066–72.
46. Penguin Project. Available at: http://penguinproject.org/. Accessed January 20, 2019.
47. Morgan's Wonderland. Available at: https://www.morganswonderland.com/. Accessed January 20, 2019.
48. University of Texas Southwestern Adaptive Sports Coalition. 2017. Available at: https://www.facebook.com/UTSWAdaptiveSports/. Accessed January 20, 2019.

Transition to Adult Care

John Berens, MD[a],*, Cynthia Wozow, DO[b], Cynthia Peacock, MD[a]

KEYWORDS

- Health care transition • Transition to adult care • Emerging adults
- Intellectual disabilities • Developmental disabilities • Chronic childhood illness
- Adolescence • Cerebral palsy

KEY POINTS

- The pediatric to adult health care transition is a challenge for many emerging adults with cerebral palsy and a structured approach is crucial to facilitate this process.
- For individuals with intellectual disabilities, it is important to consider supported decision making and partner with family members to promote optimal self-advocacy.
- There are many psychosocial considerations unique to emerging adults with cerebral palsy that are important to address during the transition process.
- There are many different opportunities for education, employment, and enrichment following high school graduation and resources exist to help individuals explore these options.
- Important changes to health insurance take place during health care transition, but several options exist to help emerging adults with cerebral palsy pay for medical care.

INTRODUCTION

Health care transition (HCT) is defined as the intentional, planned process of transferring care from a pediatric-based to adult-based health care setting. This process consists of 3 broad parts: the preparatory phase, which typically occurs in a pediatric setting; the transfer from the pediatric to adult health care setting; and the period of integration into adult-based care that follows the transfer. Nearly 5 million youth with special health care needs between the ages of 12 and 17 years will soon be eligible to transition to adult health care, which includes numerous adolescents with cerebral palsy (CP).[1] CP, the most common motor disorder of childhood, accounts for approximately 2 in 1000 live births, and about 98% of those children aged 4 to 14 years survive to age 20 years. Survival is slightly reduced for the most severely affected individuals, but this seems to be improving.[2,3] Of those who survive to age

Disclosure: The authors have nothing to disclose.
[a] Department of Internal Medicine, Section of Transition Medicine, Baylor College of Medicine, Transition Medicine Clinic, 7200 Cambridge Street, Suite 8A, Houston, TX 77030, USA;
[b] Department of Physical Medicine and Rehabilitation, Baylor College of Medicine, Texas Children's Hospital, 6701 Fannin Street, Wallace Tower 1280, Houston, TX 77030, USA
* Corresponding author.
E-mail address: john.berens@bcm.edu

Phys Med Rehabil Clin N Am 31 (2020) 159–170
https://doi.org/10.1016/j.pmr.2019.09.004
1047-9651/20/© 2019 Elsevier Inc. All rights reserved.

20 years, approximately 86% survive to age 50 years (compared with 96% in the general population),[4] although the percentage is lower for those with intellectual disability (ID), nonambulatory status, and poor manual dexterity.[5,6] With such a large proportion of these individuals living well into adulthood, HCT is a reality eventually encountered by most children born with CP.

HCT is established as a national health care priority by prominent medical societies, but available data continue to show shortcomings in the care and support received by individuals and their caregivers during this period.[7] Numerous barriers hinder successful HCTs at the level of the patient, medical provider, and medical system that have been echoed by people with CP and by the pediatric multidisciplinary providers who often serve them.[8,9] The framework of care delivery often changes from a more integrated, multidisciplinary approach to a spoke-and-wheel approach of a primary care physician and subspecialists.[10] These barriers, combined with the developmental challenges normally faced by adolescents and young adults, make this a high-risk period that is often associated with negative health outcomes.[1,7] It is important for medical providers who care for individuals with CP to be knowledgeable about the issues faced as they transition to adult-based health care. This article explores some of the most common and pertinent topics and provides relevant resources whenever possible.

SUPPORTED DECISION MAKING

On turning 18 years old, a person becomes a legal adult with the right to make independent decisions. This shift in responsibility can be difficult, especially in the case of ID, in which caregivers often play a more active role in decision making. Approximately 45% of individuals with CP have ID, although this varies by motor function (the number increases to 83% in Gross Motor Function Classification System levels IV–V) and type of motor dysfunction (more common for dyskinesia and hypotonia compared with spasticity).[6] Note also that there may be a discordance between a person's intellectual functioning and communication abilities, because 9% of people with CP and no ID are nonverbal. For individuals with severe dysarthria, it can be difficult to adequately assess intellectual functioning. An evaluation for augmentative/alternative communication systems may be considered to facilitate patient communication and, in doing so, help elucidate cognitive ability.[11]

Legal options exist for individuals with ID who require support in making decisions or managing their affairs. In most states, there are various levels of support. The most restrictive option is guardianship, in which a person (a relative, close friend, or in some cases a person appointed by the court system) is designated to make decisions on behalf of the individual who is deemed to not have the capacity to do so. In this case, capacity is typically assessed by a physician who takes into account the underlying medical diagnoses as they relate to the person's abilities and the supports that are required. Guardianship can be complete, meaning all domains are managed by the guardian, or partial, in which the individual retains independence in certain areas (eg, financial). In addition to completing the capacity evaluation, physicians often serve as a source of up-to-date information and support for their patients and caregivers. Applying for guardianship can be labor intensive and expensive, and some medical institutions have medical-legal partnerships that can provide assistance.

When considering supported decision making, it is imperative to identify the least restrictive means that ensures adequate support while not encroaching on the individual's autonomy. Some states offer a less restrictive option called shared decision making. This option does not remove legal rights but officially recognizes a chosen confidant as someone who helps the individual make decisions in 1 or more areas. Additional resources on this topic are listed in **Table 1**.

PSYCHOSOCIAL CONSIDERATIONS

Chronic medical conditions notwithstanding, the period of emerging adulthood (typically referring to ages 18–25 years) is often a time of many transitions, personal growth, and identity exploration that brings both exciting opportunities and significant challenges.[12] This period can be accompanied by many psychosocial issues that may be difficult to discuss for both patient and provider, but have a major impact on the person's health, well-being, and ability to engage in self-care. For medical providers, it is important to have a thoughtful and systematic approach to engage emerging adults in discussion on several crucial areas. Although many different standardized approaches exist, a commonly used mnemonic is the HEADSSS (home environment, education/employment/eating, activities [hobbies], drugs, sexuality, suicide/depression, and safety) examination.[13]

In order to build trust and ensure patient comfort when discussing such sensitive topics, it is important to consider who is present during these discussions, because patients may not be comfortable disclosing certain information with parents or caregivers present. Significant cognitive, behavioral, and communication issues notwithstanding, asking patients who they want to be present can foster a sense of independence and may help enrich the patient-physician relationship.

Mental Health

There is growing evidence that suggests youth with chronic health conditions experience higher rates of mental health issues compared with their peers. One study reported nearly half of all youth with anxiety also had a coexisting chronic illness; another showed that depression tends to be more severe for those with concurrent chronic illness and worsens around the transition period.[14,15] CP is no exception, because studies estimate 39% of adults with CP meet the diagnostic criteria for anxiety and 17% to 20% for depression,[16,17] and this may not have a strong relation to the patient's ambulatory status.[18] Theories to explain the increase in mental health diagnoses include prolonged exposure to increased levels of stress or a sense of increased burden and learned helplessness. It may also be related to increasing difficulties with pain, poor sleep, fatigue, and relationships[17]; relationships seem to be a protective factor for overall quality of life.[19] In a population whose physical requirements often overshadow mental health needs, it is imperative to screen for mental health disorders. This requirement is also in line with broader guidelines that recommend screening all adults for depression.[20] Recognition of these problems before transitioning to adult care can ensure they are incorporated into the overall transition plan and not forgotten among the numerous other competing issues during this period.

Sexuality and Sexual Health

As individuals with CP mature and become more aware of their diagnosis and its effect on their daily function, they may also desire to understand the impact of CP on sexuality and reproduction, with 1 study suggesting 90% of community-dwelling people with CP desire more sexual education.[21] It is important that physicians

Table 1
Resources for health care transition. Resources relevant to issues commonly encountered during the transition from pediatric-based to adult-based health care for individuals with CP.

Resource	Description	Location
Association for Driver Rehabilitation Specialists	List of driving fact sheets for various disabilities, including information on finding a local driver rehabilitation specialist	https://www.aded.net/page/510
Association of University Centers on Disabilities, postsecondary education Web page	List of resources on postsecondary education and relevant national policies	https://www.aucd.org/template/page.cfm?id=509
Employer Assistance and Resource Network on Disability Inclusion	List of state-based vocational rehabilitation agencies	http://www.askearn.org/state-vocational-rehabilitation-agencies/
Got Transition	Provides structured processes and resources surrounding HCT geared toward patients and medical providers, including reimbursement strategies	http://www.gottransition.org/
Medicaid Waivers	Link to state-based Medicaid waiver programs	http://medicaidwaiver.org/
National Resource Center for Supported Decision-Making	Resource hub and state-based list of supported decision-making options	http://supporteddecisionmaking.org/
Supplemental Security Income	Additional information regarding SSI benefits	https://www.ssa.gov/benefits/ssi/
The Arc	A national advocacy organization that serves people with intellectual and developmental disabilities and their families	https://www.thearc.org
Think College	Search and comparison tools for postsecondary education for students with intellectual disabilities	https://thinkcollege.net/college-search
Ticket to Work	Federal program facilitating employment for those receiving disability benefits; includes information on retaining Medicaid while working	https://choosework.ssa.gov/index.html
TransCen	National organization providing resources and support in finding employment for individuals with disabilities	https://www.transcen.org/

provide age-appropriate sexual education regardless of disability. The position statement on sexuality from The Arc, a national advocacy group for individuals with intellectual and developmental disabilities, emphasizes the inherent right of all people to "exercise choices regarding sexual expression and social relationships."[22] Nevertheless, factors such as increased dependence on family for daily activities, being viewed as someone needing protection, and an overall feeling of undesirability can make it increasingly difficult for patients to promote their sexual identity and intimate relationships.[23,24]

Compared with age-matched peers, individuals with CP reach sexual milestones at an older age, mostly occurring during emerging adulthood.[23] Despite 80% of young adults reporting physical issues with sex related to CP, when surveyed in a rehabilitation setting, 90% reported that it had not been discussed.[24] Issues such as incontinence, decreased sensation, and the most commonly reported concern, spasticity, are all possibly modifiable with medical treatment. As such, it is important for physicians to consider how medical conditions and physical limitations may affect romantic relationships when discussing a patient's sexual history; these concerns are well aligned with the broader goal in rehabilitation medicine of optimizing function and quality of life. In addition to these population-specific considerations, providers should be familiar with general recommendations for preventive care, including screening for sexually transmitted infections and cervical cancer, as well as related topics such as consent, fertility, and contraception. These discussions often take place in the primary care environment with involvement of specialists such as obstetrics/gynecology and urology as appropriate.

In addition, medical providers need to be aware of patients' vulnerability to sexual abuse. Individuals with developmental disabilities are at an increased risk of abuse because they are often more dependent on others for care, exposed to larger numbers of caregivers, may have poorer judgment on which behaviors are considered inappropriate, and may be less able to report abuse. The National Center on Child Abuse and Neglect reports that children and adolescents with disabilities are at a 2.2 times higher risk of sexual abuse than their peers; the lifetime risk of sexual assault for women with developmental disabilities is 68% to 83%, and only half of these cases are reported.[25] It is important for medical providers to have open, honest discussions with their patients and caregivers about these issues.

Substance Use

Experimentation with drugs and alcohol is a common but potentially high-risk behavior often seen during adolescent development. Its incidence increases with age and is influenced by many factors, including low socioeconomic status, anxiety, depression, and a greater need to "fit in." The presence of chronic illness does not seem to be a protective factor because individuals with a chronic condition are more likely to participate in risk-taking behaviors than their peers[26]; however, 1 study evaluating community-dwelling adults with CP showed lower rates of substance abuse and sexually transmitted disease.[16] For individuals with chronic illness requiring multiple medications, such as many individuals with CP, there are additional considerations when counseling on these issues. For example, alcohol may have an additive effect with certain medications (eg, baclofen or benzodiazepines) or may alter medication metabolism; additionally, alcohol may lower the seizure threshold for people with known seizure disorders.

HEALTH INSURANCE

There are often substantial changes to health insurance that occur during the HCT period. Most notably, adult-based health insurance may provide less benefits, particularly for on-going therapies (eg, physical therapy) and durable medical equipment (DME), both of which are commonly used by individuals with CP. This change may explain why 1 survey-based study in France showed significantly lower use of certain therapies, equipment, and physical medicine and rehabilitation care in adults with CP compared with children.[27] In addition, for patients receiving Supplemental Security Income (SSI; supplemental income given to individuals with eligible disabilities), there is a requalification process at age 18 years. Unlike SSI for children, parental income is no longer a factor for adult SSI, but income earned by the individual is counted, so careful planning and counseling is important for individuals who receive SSI that are considering employment.

At present, young adults in the United States may have several options available for health insurance coverage, which can include:

1. Remaining on their parents' health insurance plan through age 26 years. Most states allow coverage to extend past this age if the individual has the designation of a disabled adult with supporting documentation from a physician.
2. Coverage through a Medicaid plan. In states where Medicaid has been expanded, any individuals who are beneath certain income requirements qualify for Medicaid. In all states, individuals who receive SSI benefits automatically qualify for Medicaid. Once a person receives Medicaid, it is possible to remain on the insurance plan even if future income (to a certain extent) results in a loss of SSI, but this requires considerable advanced planning. See **Table 1** for more information on government-based insurance and benefits.
3. Coverage under their parents' established Medicare plan for individuals on SSI. Alternatively, if individuals qualify for Social Security Disability Insurance (SSDI), they then qualify for Medicare after receiving these benefits for at least 2 years. Eligibility for SSDI depends on the person's age; time employed when Social Security taxes were paid; and, most importantly, a disability preventing gainful employment. Unlike SSI, the person's assets are not a factor.
4. Purchasing health insurance on the public exchange that was initially created through the Affordable Care Act in 2010. These plans vary in cost and coverage benefits.
5. Temporary continuation of a prior employer-sponsored insurance plan through the Consolidated Omnibus Budget Reconciliation Act (COBRA) program, but only following certain life events, such as job termination.

In addition to health insurance, Medicaid waivers are another important part of comprehensive coverage for many individuals with CP. Historically, certain Medicaid services could only be provided if the person was institutionalized, but, with the shift toward deinstitutionalization of persons with disabilities, new programs waived this requirement. The goal of waiver programs is to provide benefits that allow individuals to reside in their communities. Each state has 1 or more distinct waiver programs, each with its own eligibility requirements and benefits, but in general they should be considered for persons with significant disease burden, disability, and/or large DME or nursing needs. Early discussion of waiver programs should be considered because some states have a substantial wait time to begin receiving these services, sometimes as long as 5 to 10 years. Please refer to **Table 1** for additional resources on this topic.

EDUCATION AND EMPLOYMENT

Another important transition that occurs in late adolescence and emerging adulthood is the completion of secondary school and the beginning of employment or additional education. This shift is an important developmental step that confers a sense of independence. Individuals with CP often share these goals but may face additional challenges and barriers in order to achieve them. Although employment rates are fairly stable over time, individuals with CP have a lower employment rate (estimates vary between 25% and 55%) compared with the 80% employment rate of the general population.[28,29] Similarly, rates of postsecondary education are significantly less. Compared with 40% enrollment in a 2-year or 4-year program for all individuals 18 to 24 years old, 1 study showed that less than 18% of individuals with CP had more than a high school education when they first used vocational rehabilitation services; because less than 10% of the study population had ID, this is likely an overestimate.[30,31]

Transportation

One of the most significant barriers by adults with disabilities is transportation. Despite improvements following the implementation of the Americans with Disabilities Act (ADA), individuals with disabilities account for approximately 40% of Americans without adequate transportation.[32] These limitations may be more pronounced in rural areas with scarcer public transportation options. The most commonly reported form of public transport used by people with disabilities is the bus (74%), followed by taxi, subway services, and other modalities.[32] Although standard routes and schedules may allow better planning of daily activates, there are still significant barriers to using public transportation for individuals with mobility issues. Advanced planning and early preparation with gradually increasing independence may be useful in improving confidence with, and knowledge of, the public transit system.

Along with improvements to the fixed-route public transportation system, ADA guidelines also instituted a complementary paratransit service for individuals who cannot access fixed routes. Paratransit services allow eligible individuals to request transport services for the following day as long as their origins and destinations are within 1.2 km (0.75 miles) of a fixed route. To qualify for this service, applicants must submit an application through the city of residence, complete an interview, and provide supporting medical documentation. This service expands the available options, but, like the public transport system, may still have significant limitations for people with severe communication and/or mobility impairments.

For individuals who may be able to drive, a driver rehabilitation specialist can assist with independent driving options that use adaptive equipment and modified vehicles. Local specialists can be found through resources such as the Association for Driver Rehabilitation Specialists. Please see **Table 1** for additional transportation resources.

Accommodations and Postsecondary Education

Throughout primary and secondary education, necessary accommodations are provided through a 504 plan or an Individualized Education Program. These accommodations are a guaranteed part of public education and, if a formal evaluation is not initiated by the school, parents may request one at any time. In contrast, postsecondary education does not have such an easily defined process. Most colleges and universities have an office of disabilities services that complies with section 504 under the Rehabilitation Act of 1973. These services can usually be identified on an educational institution's Web site, but accommodations typically must be requested by the individual. They may include assistance outside of general education needs such as housing and parking. An application with supporting documentation from a medical provider is often required. Please see **Table 1** for additional resources on education and related disability rights.

If an individual chooses postsecondary education, it is also important to consider the location of the educational institution. If it is remote from the current medical team, it may be necessary to collaborate with local physicians and dedicate more time developing a portable medical summary. Although it is always good practice to evaluate patient abilities related to health care independence, such as making doctor appointments, ordering medication refills, and understanding the patient's health conditions, it is especially prudent to assess these skills before patient relocation in order to ensure that adequate supports are in place.

Employment

For individuals seeking to enter the workforce, the fear of disclosing limitations can be intimidating, but the Americans with Disabilities and Rehabilitation Act forbids discrimination against those with a disability within the workforce. It also requires that employers provide reasonable accommodations unless it causes an undue hardship to the employer. A reasonable accommodation is considered to be any change in the work environment to help the person perform the duties of the job, such as wheelchair accessibility or augmentative devices.[33] Individuals with disabilities entering the workforce may benefit from local vocational rehabilitation services. These programs help secure employment through services such as vocational counseling, trade certification, on-the-job training, aid in job placement, and help with transportation (including vehicle modifications). In order to qualify for this service, the person must have a physical or mental impairment that hinders employment, as long as the disability is not so severe that employment would not be possible even with assistance. Please see **Table 1** for state-based and national resources.

Considerations for Individuals with Intellectual Disability

Planning for life after secondary school is equally important for individuals with ID. Under the Individuals with Disabilities Education Act, special education services are required to be available through the age of 21 years. On graduation, additional education or employment may be considered with appropriate supports in place. Individuals with more severe intellectual disabilities may consider attending daytime habilitation (dayhab) programs that provide peer interactions, offer developmentally appropriate activities, provide a structured schedule, and can serve as caregiver respite.

TRANSITION PLANNING

As previously discussed in this article, emerging adults with CP may experience substantial changes in their levels of independence, living situation, health insurance, and how their day-to-day lives are spent. Along with typical developmental factors and complex psychosocial considerations, this period is one of many challenges that greatly affect the transition from pediatric-based to adult-based health care. However, there are resources for medical providers that offer guidance on how to improve the 3 phases of HCT: preparation, transfer, and integration into adult-based care. Got Transition describes 6 core elements to the HCT process and provides free resources for individuals, their families/caregivers, and medical providers/clinics who care for transitioning patients.[34] There are several iterations of these tools to include situations in which there are 2 totally separate health care systems or when there is no physical transfer, such as someone continuing to see the same family physician as an adult.

Ideally, HCT preparation begins as early as age 12 years with the discussion of a transition policy (element 1). Having a policy that spells out the expected timeline for HCT sets clear expectations and also helps lay the foundation for related conversations in future encounters. Information sharing is an important component, as shown by 1 review showing large unmet information-related needs experienced by transition-age youth with CP and their parents.[9] Element 2 recommends having a transition registry or some way to identify adolescents who are approaching the age of transfer. A registry can also serve as a platform to track an individual's progress toward being ready for transfer (element 3). Many different skills are required to optimize health care independence (eg, refilling a prescription, making a follow-up appointment), so assessing these skills can identify opportunities for education and practice. As the time for the transfer approaches, the next step is to make a transition plan (element 4). This step can include creating a medical summary, identifying adult providers, and addressing topics discussed in this article, such as health insurance and medical decision making.

Element 5 is the actual transfer of care to adult health care system; the process for this step may vary by location. One approach is to first transfer primary care, which can be effective when there is no physical transfer (family medicine or combined internal medicine/pediatrics physicians) or when there is a low level of medical complexity. For individuals with CP who also have an ID and/or have a high level of medical complexity (eg, have a tracheostomy tube or require chronic ventilation), transferring primary care first may still be the preferred option if there is an adult practice with sufficient experience in caring for individuals with complex, chronic, childhood-onset medical conditions.[35] This type of practice could be thought of as tertiary primary care, or may even be more akin to a complex care clinic for adults.[36] After establishing adult primary care, the specialty-to-specialty transitions can be facilitated. In some cases, an adult specialist is not required, such as an internist managing hypertension without nephrology consultation. In other cases, it is critical to address certain medical issues before transitioning; for example, few adult orthopedists perform surgical repair of scoliosis. Given the possibility of time-sensitive issues, it is important to map out these transfers early in the HCT process.

An alternative approach to the transfer process is a consultative model. This model could include a stand-alone clinic/outpatient consult team that facilitates the various elements of the HCT and works on health independence skill-building or an inpatient consult service that identifies emerging adults in need of HCT and communicates with an outpatient clinic.[37] In all of these approaches, it is important to involve leaders who understand both the local pediatric and adult health care systems and can facilitate communication across medical institutions to work toward the common goal of more streamlined HCTs and healthier young adults.

Element 6 represents the final part of HCT: transfer completion and integration into the adult health care system. Completing the transfer can include "closing the loop" with the pediatric team and having the patient return to the pediatrician for a final visit after establishing with an adult primary care physician. A key concept regarding integration is that the work of HCT is not finished when the transfer is complete. Emerging adulthood and many of the issues discussed in this article often continue at least into the mid-20s, if not longer, so it is equally important for adult health care providers to be aware of these issues and establish processes to address them. Measuring the success of HCT often happens in the adult health care system as well. Various outcome measures have been proposed, including population health/disease-specific guide-lines (eg, improved hemoglobin A1c level in diabetes), the experience of care (eg, improved patient satisfaction), and cost/use measures (eg, decreased emergency room visits). There have been many different interventions seeking to improve these measures, such as using a care coordinator to decrease hospital use or integrating HCT supports into the electronic health record. One systematic review suggests that having structured interventions matters more than any single, specific change.[38] Combined with a quality improvement approach targeting medical practices and health care systems, these 6 core elements can be used as guides to help build and assess the strength of structured interventions to improve the entire process of HCT.[39]

REFERENCES

1. Lebrun-Harris LA, McManus MA, Ilango SM, et al. Transition planning among US youth with and without special health care needs. Pediatrics 2018;142(4) [pii: e20180194].
2. Peterson H, Lenski M, Hidecker MJC, et al. Cerebral palsy and aging. Dev Med Child Neurol 2009;51(4):16–23.
3. Strauss D, Shavelle R, Reynolds R, et al. Survival in cerebral palsy in the last 20 years: signs of improvement? Dev Med Child Neurol 2007;49:86–92.
4. Hemming K, Hutton JL, Paroah POD. Long-term survival for a cohort of adults with cerebral palsy. Dev Med Child Neurol 2006;48:90–5.
5. Hutton JL. Outcome in cerebral palsy: life-expectancy. Paediatr Child Health 2008;18(9):419–22.
6. Reid SM, Meehan EM, Arnup SJ, et al. Intellectual disability in cerebral palsy: a population-based retrospective study. Dev Med Child Neurol 2018;60(7):687–94.
7. White PH, Cooley WC, Transitions Clinical Report Authoring Group. Supporting the health care transition from adolescence to adulthood in the medical home. Pediatrics 2018;142(5) [pii:e20182587].
8. Bolger A, Vargus-Adams J, McMahon M. Transition of care in adolescents with cerebral palsy: a survey of current practices. PM R 2017;9(3):258–64.
9. Freeman M, Stewart D, Cunningham CE, et al. Information needs of young people with cerebral palsy and their families during the transition to adulthood: a scoping review. J Transit Med 2018. https://doi.org/10.1515/jtm-2018-0003.
10. Nguyen T, Baptiste S. Innovative practice: exploring acculturation theory to advance rehabilitation from pediatric to adult "cultures" of care. Disabil Rehabil 2015;37(5):456–63.
11. Myrden A, Schudlo L, Weyand S, et al. Trends in communicative access solutions for children with cerebral palsy. J Child Neurol 2014;29(8):1108–18.
12. Arnet JJ. Emerging adulthood: a theory of development from the late teens through the twenties. Am Psychol 2000;55(5):469–80.
13. Goldenring JM, Rosen DS. Getting into adolescent heads: an essential update. Contemp Pediatr 2004;21(1):64–92.
14. Chavira DA, Garland AF, Daley S, et al. The impact of medical comorbidity on mental health and functional health outcomes among children with anxiety disorders. J Dev Behav Pediatr 2008;29:394–402.
15. Ferro MA, Gorter JW, Boyle MH. Trajectories of depressive symptoms during the transition to young adulthood: the role of chronic illness. J Affect Disord 2015;174:594–601.

16. Fortuna RJ, Holub A, Turk MA, et al. Health conditions, functional status and health care utilization in adults with cerebral palsy. Fam Pract 2018;35(6): 661–70.

17. Smith KJ, Peterson MD, O'Connell NE, et al. Risk of depression and anxiety in adults with cerebral palsy. JAMA Neurol 2018. https://doi.org/10.1001/jamaneurol.2018.4147.

18. Linhares D, Hung C, Matsumoto H, et al. The 'true' prevalence and risk factors of depression in adults with cerebral palsy. 2017. Available at: https://doi.org/10.1111/dmcn.67_13512. Accessed March 15, 2019.

19. Maestro-Gonzalez A, Bilbao-Leon MC, Zuazua-Rico D, et al. Quality of life as assessed by adults with cerebral palsy. PLoS One 2018;13(2):e0191960.

20. Siu AL, US Preventive Services Task Force. Screening for depression in adults: US preventive services task force recommendation statement. JAMA 2016; 315(4):380–7.

21. Murphy KP, Molnar GE, Lankasky K. Employment and social issues in adults with cerebral palsy. Arch Phys Med Rehabil 2000;81(6):807–11.

22. The Arc. Sexuality position statement. 2013. Available at: https://www.thearc.org/who-we-are/position-statements/life-in-the-community/sexuality. Accessed March 13, 2019.

23. Wiegerink DJ, Stam HJ, Gorter JW, et al. Development of romantic relationships and sexual activity in young adults with cerebral palsy: a longitudinal study. Arch Phys Med Rehabil 2010;91:1423–8.

24. Wiegerink D, Roebroeck M, Bender J, et al. Sexuality of young adults with cerebral palsy: experienced limitations and needs. Sex Disabil 2011;29(2):119–28.

25. Murphy NA, Elias ER, Council on Children with Disabilities. Sexuality of children and adolescents with developmental disabilities. Pediatrics 2006;118(1): 398–403.

26. Suris J, Michaud P, Akre C, et al. Health risk behaviors in adolescents with chronic conditions. Pediatrics 2008;122(5):e1113–8.

27. Roquet M, Garlantezec R, Remy-Neris O, et al. From childhood to adulthood: health care use in individuals with cerebral palsy. Dev Med Child Neurol 2018; 60:1271–7.

28. Frisch D, Msall ME. Health, functioning, and participation of adolescents and adults with cerebral palsy: a review of outcomes research. Dev Disabil Res Rev 2013;18:84–94.

29. Benner JL, Hilberink SR, Veenis T, et al. Course of employment in adults with cerebral palsy over a 14-year period. Dev Med Child Neurol 2017;59(7):762–8.

30. Huang I, Holzbauer JJ, Lee E, et al. Vocational rehabilitation services and employment outcomes for adults with cerebral palsy in the United States. Dev Med Child Neurol 2013;55(11):1000–8.

31. US department of Commerce, Census Bureau. Current population survey. 2017. Available at: https://nces.ed.gov/programs/coe/indicator_cpb.asp. Accessed March 14, 2019.

32. Bezyak JL, Sabella SA, Gattis RH. Public transportation: an investigation of barriers for people with disabilities. J Disabil Policy Stud 2017;28(1):52–60.

33. U.S. Equal Employment Opportunity Commission. Disability discrimination. 2015. Available at: https://www.eeoc.gov/laws/types/disability.cfm. Accessed March 15, 2019.

34. Got transition. Six core elements of health care transition 2.0. 2014. Available at: https://www.gottransition.org/resourceGet.cfm?id=206. Accessed March 13, 2019.

35. Berens JC, Peacock C. Implementation of an academic adult primary care clinic for adolescents and young adults with complex, chronic childhood conditions. J Pediatr Rehabil Med 2015;8:3–12.
36. Maeng DD, Snyder SR, Davis TW, et al. Impact of a complex care management model on cost and utilization among adolescents and young adults with special care and health needs. Popul Health Manag 2017;20(6):435–41.
37. Gold JI, Boudos R, Shah P, et al. Transition consultative models in two academic medical centers. Pediatr Ann 2017;46(6):e235–41.
38. Gabriel P, McManus M, Rogers K, et al. Outcome evidence for structured pediatric to adult health care transition interventions: a systematic review. J Pediatr 2017;188:263–9.
39. McManus M, White P, Barbour A, et al. Pediatric to adult transition: a quality improvement model for primary care. J Adolesc Health 2015;56:73–8.

FURTHER READINGS

Berens J, Blazo M, Peacock C. Transitioning to adult care. In: Dhar S, editor. Handbook of clinical adult genetics and genomics: a practice-based approach. Amsterdam: Elsevier; 2020.
Pilapil M, DeLaet DE, Kuo AA, et al. Care of adults with chronic childhood conditions: a practical guide. Switzerland: Springer International; 2016. p. 1–12, 67–85, 365–420.

Orthopedic Conditions in Adults with Cerebral Palsy

Megan R. Lomax, MMS, MPAS, PA-C[a], M. Wade Shrader, MD[b],*

KEYWORDS

- Adults • Cerebral palsy • Orthopedic conditions

KEY POINTS

- Orthopedic conditions in adults with cerebral palsy (CP) lead to chronic pain, skin breakdown, and decline in mobility and function.
- With more adults with CP living longer lives, new or increasing problems need to be addressed as we seek to improve quality of life in this patient population with focused treatments to decrease pain, maintain activity, and maximize function.
- Identifying goals that are realistic and attainable should be the priority of the provider when deciding to intervene with orthopedic surgery.

Cerebral palsy (CP) is the most common cause of physical disability in childhood.[1] With increasing survival of preterm infants and increasing survivorship into adulthood, the overall society prevalence continues to increase. Although the exact number is unknown, it is estimated that between 700,000 and 1 million adults in the United States have CP.[2] As children with CP transition to adulthood, they face many challenges. In addition, those with CP experience "premature aging" and tend to have a much quicker decline in mobility and walking skills as compared with otherwise healthy population.[3,4,5] Patients with functional levels, Gross Motor Function Classification System (GMFCS) levels II to V, have been shown to lose some gross motor function, as measured by GMFM.

Although CP is considered a nonprogressive condition of the brain, the musculoskeletal components tend to worsen and deteriorate over time.[6,7] Primary impairments of CP include abnormal muscle tone, loss of selective muscle control, impaired coordination and balance, weakness, and loss of sensation. These primary impairments coupled with the effects of growth, time, and developmental delays negatively affect the musculoskeletal system. Weakness and tone abnormalities may lead to progressive contractures. Persistent tone, increased body mass index, contractures, and lever arm dysfunction may lead to increased loads across joints with subsequent early arthritis and pain.

[a] Texas Children's Hospital, 6701 Fannin Street, Suite 660, Houston, TX 77030, USA; [b] Nemours A.I. duPont Hospital for Children, 1600 Rockland Road, Wilmington, DE 19807, USA
* Corresponding author.
E-mail address: Wade.shrader@nemours.org

Phys Med Rehabil Clin N Am 31 (2020) 171–183
https://doi.org/10.1016/j.pmr.2019.09.013
pmr.theclinics.com

Orthopedic care of adults with CP has not been well documented in the literature. There are few institutions in the country equipped to fully care for adults living with CP who have orthopedic issues. Orthopedic care for children with CP within the environment of children's hospitals is often appropriate until ages 16 to 21 years. Many families with children living with CP experience the "falling off the cliff" that occurs during the transition from pediatric to adult health services. With more adults with CP living longer lives, new or increasing problems need to be addressed as we seek to improve quality of life in this patient population with focused treatments to decrease pain, maintain activity, and maximize function.[5]

CHRONIC PAIN

Chronic pain due to early arthritis, especially of the neck, back, and lower extremities is relatively common in most of the adults with CP, with an estimated 25% experiencing degenerative joint disease in their 20s.[5,8] Because the joints are not experiencing full range of motion with increased joint forces due to spasticity, they tend to wear out much quicker than in the general population. Solutions to pain are multimodal and include spasticity management (botox and oral medications such as baclofen and valium), massage/chiropractic/healing touch, wheelchair modifications, and frequent changing of positions. Although pain medications are an option, substance abuse is an issue along with worsening of constipation. There may be a role of cannabinoids in the treatment of pain in people living with CP, although this must be further studied.

SPINE CONDITIONS

Neuromuscular scoliosis (**Fig. 1**) is a spine deformity that possibly has the most effect on longevity of the patient with CP. The cause of scoliosis in CP is not entirely clear, but it is thought to be due to a combination of muscle weakness, truncal imbalance, and asymmetric tone in paraspinous and intercostal muscles.[9] It is more common in GMFCS IV and V patients.[10] Unlike adolescent idiopathic scoliosis, a very high percentage of neuromuscular curves tend to severely progress with time, resulting in adverse effects on the heart and lungs, as well as leading to pelvic obliquity, which affects seating and leads to skin breakdown and decubitus ulcers. Initial treatment of neuromuscular scoliosis is typically seating and wheelchair modifications. Bracing with spine orthoses may be offered but have not been shown to be effective. Once neuromuscular curves reach 50°, they tend to rapidly progress.[11] Posterior spinal instrumentation and fusion (PSIF) is the mainstay of treatment of severe neuromuscular curves (**Fig. 2**).[2] The goals of PSIF are to straighten the spine, balance the spine and trunk, lower the risk of progression, allow for easier sitting and positioning, relieve pain, decrease other complications including decubiti and lung disease, and improve quality of life. It is typically recommended in adolescence; however, many parents hesitate to pursue surgery until obvious curve progression. Although surgery can be performed in older adults, there is a higher complication rate, especially in patients with multiple medical problems.[12] Yet, the benefits of surgery seem to outweigh the risks of complications as demonstrated through several high-quality studies published by the Harms study group.[13] In most recent years, some CP programs have moved toward systematic processes of critically evaluating patients in a multidisciplinary setting to ensure the right surgery is performed on the right patient, thereby minimizing postoperative complications.

Spinal stenosis or a narrowing of the spinal canal can lead to neurologic deficits from spinal cord compression or myopathy. The most common type of spinal stenosis in adults with CP is cervical stenosis (**Fig. 3**). Significant movement disorders such as dystonia or

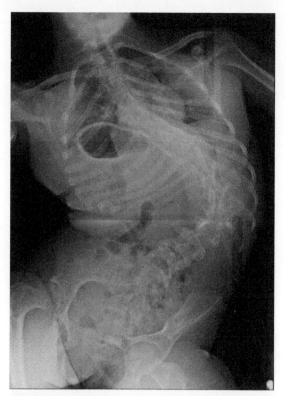

Fig. 1. Neuromuscular scoliosis. (*Courtesy of* M. Wade Shrader, MD, Wilmington, DE.)

athetosis can contribute to development of cervical myopathy due to contorsional head and neck postures. In patients with dystonic CP, there is an 8-fold increase in degenerative joint disease and instability potentially leading to radicular pain, myopathy, and neurologic deficits.[14,15] Providers should be wary of spinal stenosis in patients complaining of loss of function.[14] In patients at higher risk, serial neurologic examinations and MRIs every 2 years should be performed for surveillance.[16] Prevention through medical management of dystonia is recommended along with seating and positional modifications. Surgical decompression (anterior, possibly both) and fusion may be necessary for rapidly progressing cases, those that fail to respond to conservative treatments, and if progressive functional loss is present. Providers caring for adult patients with CP need to be aware that increased spasticity, declining motor function, and changes in bowel and bladder function may represent a myelopathic picture as opposed to a change in neurologic function simply due to aging.

Thoracic and lumbar stenoses are not as common as cervical stenosis with dystonia; however, they may be associated with progressive scoliosis, especially because what was initially an adolescent type of neuromuscular scoliosis erodes into a superimposed degenerative spine deformity. Again, this condition should be suspected in any patients with myelopathic symptoms and loss of function.[14] Conservative treatment includes nonsteroidal antiinflammatory medications, epidural injections, and physical therapy. Progressive pain and neurologic loss require surgical treatment with posterior spinal fusion and decompression.

Spondylolysis and spondylolisthesis are other common spinal conditions that affect the adult CP population. Spondylolysis is an acquired condition involving a stress

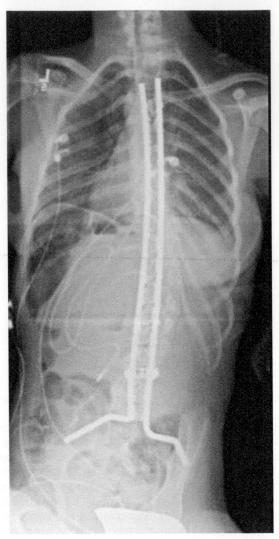

Fig. 2. Posterior spinal instrumentation and fusion. (*Courtesy of* M. Wade Shrader, MD, Wilmington, DE.)

fracture through the pars interarticularis, thought to be due to repetitive hyperextension.[17] In the general population, 6% of people are affected.[18] The prevalence is 20% among GMFCS I to III patients.[15,16,19,20] This number is higher after selective dorsal rhizotomy. Typically, spondylolysis is responsive to conservative treatment including physical therapy and activity modifications; however, progression to spondylolisthesis may require L4-S1 posterior spinal fusion.[15,16,20]

HIP CONDITIONS

Neuromuscular hip dysplasia is a significant issue in children with CP.[21] The incidence varies between 10% and 90% and increases with increasing GMFCS levels, most commonly affecting GMFCS IV and V. Untreated hip dysplasia in patients with CP

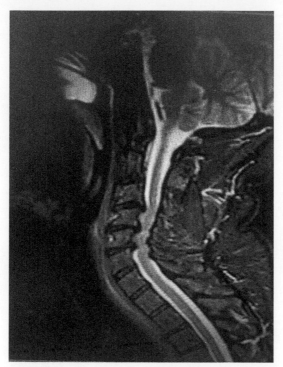

Fig. 3. Cervical stenosis. (*Courtesy of* David Frumberg, MD, New Haven, CT.)

can lead to frank dislocation (**Fig. 4**) over time due to abnormal forces acting on the femoral head. This eventually leads to degenerative joint disease (**Fig. 5**) and pain. Although young patients with hip dislocation may be asymptomatic, degenerative joint disease of the hip is the leading cause of pain in adults with CP, affecting up to 50% of adults living with CP.[22] Pain from hip degenerative joint disease can lead to severe loss of quality of life. Treatment in children is focused on preventing dislocation and reducing dislocated hips before femoral head and acetabular dysplastic changes occur. Moderately high success rates are reported in the literature, which has led to a national push for formalized hip surveillance with serial radiographs until skeletal maturity. Once hip dysplasia, hip arthritis, and pain are present, treatment options are limited to either hip salvage or reconstruction; therefore, most orthopedic surgeons are united on taking a preventative approach.[23,24]

HIP SALVAGE

Proximal femoral resection was first reported by Castle and involves an osteotomy less than the level of the lesser trochanter with interposition of the abductors sewn over the acetabulum and the vastus lateralis over the femur. This procedure is meant to eliminate the source of pain.[25,26] The McHale procedure moves the proximal femur laterally away from areas of impingement. The surgery involves removal of the femoral head ("Girdlestone" procedure) in combination with a valgus proximal femoral osteotomy.[27] These procedures are reserved for nonambulatory patients, including those who cannot crawl.[28] Although these procedures have been found to offer good pain relief, they are not without complications. Heterotopic ossification and proximal

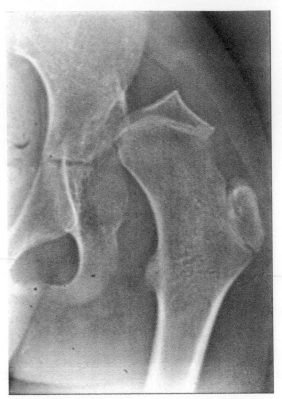

Fig. 4. Untreated hip dysplasia in patients with CP can lead to frank dislocation over time due to abnormal forces acting on the femoral head. (*Courtesy of* M. Wade Shrader, MD, Wilmington, DE.)

migration are the most commonly reported complications.[25] Both procedures have been found to provide good pain relief and improve seating and hygiene, although most studies recommend proximal femur resection due to decreased complication rates.[23,24,28,29]

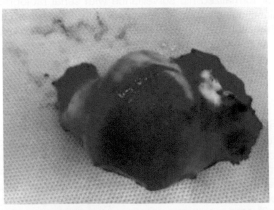

Fig. 5. Frank dislocation eventually leads to degenerative joint disease and pain. (*Courtesy of* M. Wade Shrader, MD, Wilmington, DE.)

ARTHROPLASTY

Total hip arthroplasty (**Fig. 6**) is another option for painful CP hips; however, this procedure is considered to be high risk with many pitfalls. Severely dysplastic hips may make acetabular implantation technically difficult and impossible. Nonambulatory patients with CP may have too small femurs for implants. Loosening and fractures may result from osteopenic bone leading to poor bone stock. Repeat dislocation may occur due to spasticity. Historically, there has been bias against arthroplasty in CP with few surgeons comfortable with performing the procedure in this patient population. Although less commonly performed, data do show this procedure has a high degree of patient satisfaction[30] in addition to good pain relief.[30–35]

A variation on total hip arthroplasty has been pioneered at DuPont, which involves a shoulder prosthesis interpositional arthroplasty. This procedure has been used in patients who have had a prior salvage procedure (Castle or McHale) but had recurrent hip pain. This procedure has been found to provide great relief of pain while also having high caretaker satisfaction.[35]

KNEE AND GAIT

The knee is a common source of pain and gait dysfunctions in patients with CP.[36] Most common orthopedic knee pathologies seen in adults with CP includes patella alta, knee flexion contractures, patella subluxations/dislocations, and inferior patellar pole fractures.

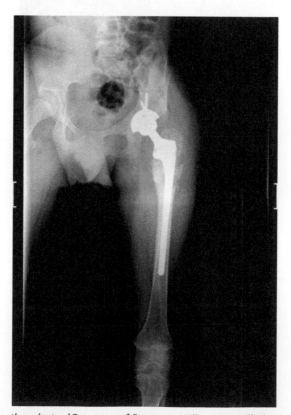

Fig. 6. Total hip arthroplasty. (*Courtesy of* Freeman Miller, MD, Wilmington, DE.)

Patella Alta and Patella Fractures

Patella alta (**Fig. 7**) is relatively common in ambulatory adults with CP. It typically begins in adolescence but progresses over time and may lead to anterior knee pain.[36] Patella alta results from quadriceps insufficiency and weakness and may progress over time. The increased strain due to the abnormal position of the patella may lead to patellar pole fractures, which are usually treated conservatively with a cast.

Hamstring Contractures and Knee Flexion Contractures

Hamstring tightness and knee flexion contractures lead to difficulty in gait for ambulators, and significant contractures can interfere with seating for non-ambulators. Botox, physical therapy, and bracing may be used to treat contractures of the hamstrings; however, fixed knee flexion contractures of greater than 10° typically need more aggressive treatment and can be treated with distal femoral extension osteotomy (DFEO) and patellar tendon advancement (tibial tubercle advancement in skeletally mature individuals). Surgical lengthening of the hamstrings may also be required. DFEO + patella tendon advancement is associated with improvement in knee positioning of stance and treatment of knee flexion contractures, but it has not been shown to necessarily improve knee pain in early adulthood.[37]

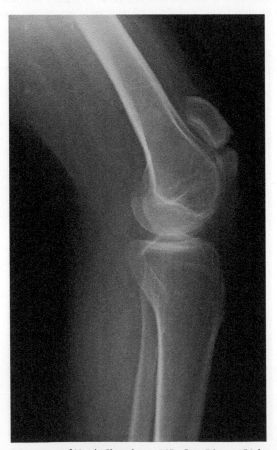

Fig. 7. Patella alta. (*Courtesy of* Hank Chambers, MD, San Diego, CA.)

BONY MALALIGNMENT

Other bony abnormalities occasionally seen in patients with CP include miserable malalignment, genu varum, and genu valgum. "Miserable malalignment" syndrome involves increased femoral anteversion and external tibial torsion, which may require femoral and tibial derotational osteotomies. Genu varum and genu valgum may lead to chronic injuries of the cruciate ligaments. Orthopedic treatment involves wedge osteotomies to improve overall limb alignment. Additional knee problems in adults with CP include meniscal tears and tricompartmental arthritis, just as occurs with adults with no neurologic disorders. Joint replacement is an option for knee deformities, especially in unreconstructable patellar-femoral deformities.

In the pediatric CP population, single-event multilevel surgery (SEMLS) is the mainstay of treatment of crouch gait. SEMLS has been used in the adult population, although there are few published studies. In theory, the principles would be similar with one surgery and one comprehensive rehabilitation versus staged procedures; however, access to prolonged rehab may be more difficult for adults, but extended rehabilitation is necessary when significant lower extremity surgery is being performed. In addition, patients had worse outcomes if they had had prior history of SEMLS as a child.[38] If multilevel orthopedic surgery is considered, gait analysis can be performed for patients to evaluate the rotational malalignment of the tibia and femur.

FOOT AND ANKLE CONDITIONS

Foot and ankle deformities in adults with CP are similar in nature to those in the pediatric population; however, contractures and deformity tend to be much rigid and less responsive to soft tissue management.[7,39] These issues lead to difficulty with shoe wear, pain, and contribute to walking decline. Treatment goals differ among ambulatory and nonambulatory patients. In ambulatory patients, treatment is focused on providing stability for ambulation and function, preventing pain and further deformity. In the nonambulatory patient, having a braceable and pain-free foot is of utmost importance. The following are the common orthopedic deformities found in an adult patient with CP.

Equinus

Equinus is the most common type of foot and ankle deformity in the CP population. It is due to a shortened achilles and gastrocnemius/soleus complex tightness. Initial treatment of stretching and/or botox may be tried in adults but is not typically successful in a real contracture. Surgical treatment involves either lengthening of the fascia or tendoachilles lengthening. Types of fascial lengthening include the Strayer, Baker, or Vulpius techniques. Equinus alone is rarely seen in the adult CP population and typically found in combination with varus and valgus foot deformities as discussed later.

Calcaneus

Calcaneus deformity or pointing upward of the foot is usually iatrogenic in nature due to overlengthening of the achilles. Nonoperative treatment includes the use of floor reaction orthosis. Surgical treatment includes muscle transfers to the heel, heel cord tenodesis, and a calcaneal osteotomy with or without muscle transfer, but none of these procedures are highly effective. The best treatment of calcaneus deformity is prevention by not overlengthening Achilles tendons in children with CP.

Equinovarus

Varus deformity is the inward curvature of the heel. Equinovarus deformity is common in those with hemiplegia. Rigid deformities place stress on the lateral aspect of the foot, causing callosities and pain.[39] Surgical treatment options include the following: frost lengthening of the posterior tibialis muscle, split posterior tibialis tendon transfer, split anterior tibialis tendon transfer, Multiple osteotomies of the foot, including calcaneal, cuboid, cuneiform, and first metatarsal, and triple arthrodesis are more typically indicated in adults with CP due to the usual rigid deformities.

Equinovalgus

Equinovalgus deformity of the foot is most commonly seen in diplegia and quadriplegia. Often called the "flatfoot," it is commonly associated with midfoot break. Treatment options for the valgus foot include peroneal brevis tendon lengthening (with other procedures), calcaneal lengthening, subtalar arthrodesis, talonavicular arthrodesis, and triple arthrodesis.

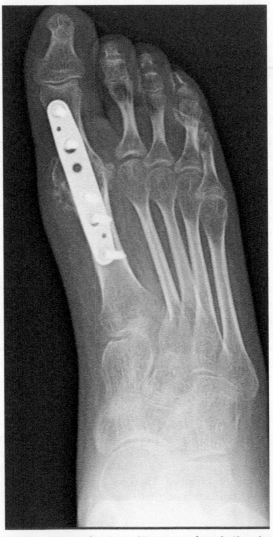

Fig. 8. Orthopedic surgery to treat bunions. (*Courtesy of* Hank Chambers, MD, San Diego, CA.)

Bunion deformities

Dorsal bunion and hallux valgus are 2 types of bunion deformities common in adults with CP, affecting the first metatarsophalangeal joint and potentially leading to pain and difficulty with shoewear. Orthopedic surgery to treat bunions aims to improve stability by fusing the joint (**Fig. 8**).

SUMMARY

In the pediatric population, orthopedic surgery to treat neuromuscular foot and ankle deformities typically involves muscle lengthening and transfers or a combination of those with correction of bony deformities through osteotomies. In adults, tendon lengthening at the ankle may not have much of an effect. Osteotomies are often necessary but may not be powerful enough to correct the magnitude of the deformity. Arthrodesis can and should be used more frequently.[7,39]

DISCUSSION/SUMMARY

In the end, identifying goals that are realistic and attainable should be the priority of the provider. It is paramount to take into consideration the functional status of the patient and to prioritize which orthopedic procedures will allow them to maintain and maximize function over time.

Who should perform orthopedic surgery on adults with CP is a difficult question. Most adult orthopedic providers do not have experience with adults with neuromuscular disabilities. Adult health care facilities also typically struggle with patients with CP, especially those with a co-existing intellectual disability. Many families are much more comfortable in a pediatric health care environment. However, some adults with CP have significant "adult medical issues" that pediatric providers and hospitals (PICU for example) do not have experience, either. It is a difficult situation.

For spine procedures, spine fusions for scoliosis up to age 25 to 30 can typically be done in either a pediatric or adult environment. The experience of the surgeon and the acceptiveness of the institution, especially the hospitalists and the ICU physicians are the most important factors. Once patients are older than 30 or if there are surgical needs for complex spine surgical techniques, such as neural decompressions or cervical spine instrumentation, then the care of an adult spine expert is probably best.

The issue of hip surgery is also complex. Pediatric orthopedic surgeons have the most experience with salvage procedures, but typically have little recent arthroplasty experience. Adult arthroplasty surgeons are technical experts in the procedure, but hardly ever take care of patients with CP. The ideal scenario is a team approach that is common in some university or tertiary care facilities where both the pediatric orthopedists and the adult arthroplasty surgeon are involved with the care. The pediatric surgeon can help with soft tissue management and postoperative tone management, and the arthroplasy surgeon can perform a technically difficult joint replacement even in the face of significant anatomic challenges.

Foot and ankle surgery is the most common lower extremity surgical need in adults with CP. Those procedures are commonly performed by adult foot and ankle specialists. The ability to consult with a CP expert to assist in decision making and patient selection can help improve surgical judgment for the adult foot and ankle expert seeing adults with CP.

DISCLOSURE STATEMENT

The authors have nothing to disclose.

REFERENCES

1. Kuban KC, Allred EN, O'Shea M, et al. An algorithm for identifying and classifying cerebral palsy in young children. J Pediatr 2008;153(4):466–72.
2. Goldstein, CPIR Foundation Scientific Advisory Council.
3. Morgan P, McGinley J. Gait function and decline in adults with cerebral palsy: a systematic review. Disabil Rehabil 2014;36(1):1–9.
4. Jahnsen R, Villien L, Egeland T, et al. Locomotion skills in adults with cerebral palsy. Clin Rehabil 2004;18(3):309–16.
5. Benner JL, Hilbrerink SR, Veenis T, et al. Long-term deterioration of perceived health and functioning in adults with cerebral palsy. Arch Phys Med Rehabil 2017;98:2196–205.
6. Turk MA, Scandale J, Rosenbaum PF, et al. The health of women with cerebral palsy. Phys Med Rehabil Clin N Am 2001;12(1):153–68.
7. Horstmann HM, Hosalkar H, Keenan MA. Orthopedic issues in the musculoskeletal care of adults with cerebral palsy. Dev Med Child Neurol 2009;51(Supl 4): 99–105.
8. Van Der Slot WA, Niouwenhuijsen C, Van Den Berg-Emons RJ, et al. Chronic pain, fatigue, and depressive symptoms in adults with spastic bilateral cerebral palsy. Dev Med Child Neurol 2012;54(9):836–42.
9. Imrie MN, Yaszay B. Management of spinal deformity in cerebral palsy. Orthop Clin North Am 2010;41(4):531–47.
10. Morell DS, Pearson JM, Sauser DD. Progressive bone and joint abnormalities of the spine and lower extremities in cerebral palsy. Radiographics 2002;22(2): 257–68.
11. Thometz JG, Simon SR. Progression of scoliosis after skeletal maturity in institutionalized adults who have cerebral palsy. J Bone Joint Surg Am 1988;70(9): 1290–6.
12. Lonstein JE, Koop SE, Novacheck TF, et al. Results and complications after spinal fusion for neuromuscular scoliosis in cerebral palsy and static encephalopathy using luque Galveston instrumentation: experience in 93 patients. Spine 2012; 37(7):583–91.
13. Miyanji F, Nasto LA, Sponseller PD, et al. Assessing the risk-benefit ratio of scoliosis surgery in cerebral palsy. J Bone Joint Surg Am 2018;100(7):556–63.
14. Fuji T, Yonenbu K, Fukiwara K, et al. Cervical radiculopathy or myelopathy secondary to athetoid cerebral palsy. J Bone Joint Surg Am 1987;69(6):815–21.
15. Harada T, Ebara S, Anwar MM, et al. The cervical spine in athetoid cerebral palsy. A radiological study of 180 patients. J Bone Joint Surg Br 1996;78(4):613–9.
16. Murphy KP. Cerebral palsy lifetime care – four musculoskeletal conditions. Dev Med Child Neurol 2009;51(Suppl. 4):30–7.
17. Able MF. Orthopedic knowledge update. Rosemont (IL): American Academy of Orthopedic Surgeons; 2006.
18. Fredrickson BE, Baker D, McHolick WJ, et al. The natural history of spondylosis and spondylolisthesis. J Bone Joint Surg Am 1984;66(5):699–707.
19. Sakai T, Yamada H, Nakamura T, et al. Lumbar spinal disorders in patients with athetoid cerebral palsy: a clinical and biomechanical study. Spine 2006;31(3): E66–70.
20. Henrikus WL, Rosenthal RK, Kasser JR. Incidence of spondylolisthesis in ambulatory cerebral palsy patients. J Pediatr Orthop 1993;13(1):37–40.
21. Soo B, Howard JJ, Boyd RN, et al. Hip displacement in cerebral palsy. J Bone Joint Surg Am 2006;88(1):121–9.

22. Hodgkinson I, Jindrich ML, Duhaut P, et al. Hip pain in 234 non-ambulatory adolescents and young adults with cerebral palsy: a cross-sectional multicenter study. Dev Med Child Neurol 2001;43(12):806–8.
23. Hwang JH, Varte L, Kim HW, et al. Salvage procedures for the painful chronically dislocated hip in cerebral palsy. Bone Joint J 2016;98-B(1):137–43.
24. Boldingh EJ, Bouwhuis CB, Van der Heijden-Maessen HC, et al. Palliative hip surgery in severe cerebral palsy: a systematic review. J Pediatr Orthop B 2014;23(1):86–92.
25. McCarthy RE, Simon S, Douglas B, et al. Proximal femoral resection to allow adults who have severe cerebral palsy to sit. J Bone Joint Surg Am 1998;70:1011–6.
26. Castle ME, Schenider C. Proximal femoral resection-interposition arthroplasty. J Bone Joint Surg Am 1978;60(8):1051–4.
27. McHale KA, Bagg M, Nason SS. Treatment of the chronically dislocated hip in adolescents with cerebral palsy with femoral head resection and subtrochanteric valgus osteotomy. J Pediatr Orthop 1990;10(4):504–9.
28. Patel NK, Sabharwal S, Gooding CR, et al. Proximal femoral excision with interposition myoplasty for cerebral palsy patients with painful chronic hip dislocation. J Child Orthop 2015;9(4):263–71.
29. Dartnell J, Gough M, Paterson JM, et al. Proximal femoral resection without postoperative traction for the painful dislocated hip in young patients with cerebral palsy: a review of 79 cases. Bone Joint J 2014;96-B(5):701–6.
30. King G, Hunt LP, Wilkinson JM, et al. Good outcome of total hip replacement in patients with cerebral palsy. Acta Orthop 2016;87(2):93–9.
31. Schroeder K, Hauck C, Wledenhofer B, et al. Long-term results of hip arthroplasty in ambulatory patients with cerebral palsy. Int Orthop 2010;34(3):335–9.
32. Raphael BS, Dines JS, Akerman M, et al. Long-term followup of total hip arthroplasty in patients with cerebral palsy. Clin Orthop Relat Res 2010;468(7):1845–54.
33. Morin C, Ursu C, Delecourt C. Total hip replacement in young non-ambulatory cerebral palsy patients. Orthop Traumatol Surg Res 2016;103(7):845–9.
34. Houdek MT, Watts CD, Wyles CC, et al. Total hip arthroplasty in patients with cerebral palsy: a cohort study matched to patients with osteoarthritis. J Bone Joint Surg Am 2017;99(6):488–93.
35. Gabos PG, Miller F, Galban MA, et al. Prosthetic interposition arthroplasty for palliative treatment of end-stage spastic hip disease in nonambulatory patients with cerebral palsy. J Pediatr Orthop 1999;19(6):796–804.
36. Senaran H, Holden C, Dabney KW, et al. Anterior knee pain in children with cerebral palsy. J Pediatr Orthop 2007;27:12–6.
37. Boyer ER, Stout JL, Laine JC, et al. Long-term outcomes of distal femoral extension osteotomy and patellar tendon advancement in individuals with cerebral palsy. J Bone Joint Surg Am 2018;100:31–41.
38. Putz C, Doderlein L, Mertens EM, et al. Multilevel surgery in adults with cerebral palsy. Bone Joint J 2016;98-B(2):282–8.
39. Karamitopoulos MS, Nirenstein L. Neuromuscular foot spastic cerebral palsy. Foot Ankle Clin 2015;20(4):657–68.

Registry-based Research in Cerebral Palsy

The Cerebral Palsy Research Network

Edward A. Hurvitz, MD[a],*, Paul H. Gross[b],
Mary E. Gannotti, PT, PhD[c], Amy F. Bailes, PT, PhD[d],
Susan D. Horn, PhD[e]

KEYWORDS

- Cerebral palsy • Registry • Cerebral palsy research network
- Comparative effectiveness research

KEY POINTS

- A national, center-based cerebral palsy registry has been built by the Cerebral Palsy Research Network to facilitate comparative effectiveness research using practice-based evidence.
- A patient-centered research agenda for cerebral palsy highlighted the need for the longitudinal studies of aging, exercise, and the comparative effectiveness of interventions.
- A multicenter registry and network can enable the development of learning health systems to improve outcomes in cerebral palsy.

Cerebral palsy (CP) is one of the most common pediatric onset physical disorders, with an incidence of approximately 3 per 1000 births.[1] There is a robust community of researchers working on questions related to CP, including earlier diagnosis, effectiveness of interventions, harnessing neuroplasticity, and long-term outcomes. The heterogeneous nature of CP, however, precludes any one center from having access to enough subjects to perform studies with sufficient power to answer critical questions, such as comparative effectiveness or long-term outcomes of interventions, or

Disclosure Statement: The authors have nothing to disclose.
[a] Department of Physical Medicine and Rehabilitation, Michigan Medicine/University of Michigan, 325 East Eisenhower Parkway, Ann Arbor, MI 48108, USA; [b] Department of Population Health Sciences, University of Utah, 295 Chipeta Way, Williams Building, Salt Lake City, UT 84108, USA; [c] Department of Rehabilitation Sciences, University of Hartford, Dana 401F, 200 Bloomfield Avenue, West Hartford, CT 06117, USA; [d] Division of Occupational Therapy and Physical Therapy, Cincinnati Children's Hospital Medical Center, 3333 Burnet Avenue, MLC 4007, Cincinnati, OH 45229, USA; [e] Health System Innovation and Research Division, Department of Population Health Sciences, University of Utah School of Medicine, Williams Building, Room 1N474, 295 Chipeta Way, Salt Lake City, UT 84108, USA
* Corresponding author.
E-mail address: ehurvitz@umich.edu

Phys Med Rehabil Clin N Am 31 (2020) 185–194
https://doi.org/10.1016/j.pmr.2019.09.005
1047-9651/20/© 2019 Elsevier Inc. All rights reserved.

establish best practices for various subtypes of CP. Multisite research is required to accomplish these goals. This type of research, however, is difficult and expensive when it is approached by groups of investigators reinventing small networks of a few centers for individual studies. The solution to this problem is to create a network of centers with established infrastructure in place to facilitate investigations with a registry of patients whose data can help answer these questions.

There are several different kind of registries. They include population registries, which gather data on all or most of the members of a given population, generally defined geographically. Population-based registries are created with the support of national or regional health care systems. These registries allow for robust studies of incidence, prevalence, and risk factors,[2] and they eliminate the bias of clinic based registries toward individuals with medical problems, geographic access, those with insurance, and other factors. Most CP registries are clinical registries, which include patients who are brought into the registry system through their attendance of clinics or through dissemination of the registry into the community to obtain volunteers. Clinical registries may be based on health condition (eg, CP and spina bifida); health services received (eg, surgical procedure and access to telemedicine/teletherapy); or particular product (eg, intrathecal baclofen pump or a particular medication).[3] A recent review found more than 150 major clinical registries in the United States.[4] Clinical registries for CP in the United States include Shriners Health Outcomes Network, which gathers data on CP and other conditions from Shriners hospitals; the Cerebral Palsy Research Registry, based at Northwestern University in Chicago, which is designed to connect investigators with potential research subjects as well as to gather patient-reported clinical information; and the Cerebral Palsy Research Network (CPRN) registry, described in detail in this article. Several large centers have their own databases, such as the Weinberg Family Cerebral Palsy Center in New York, which has more than 4000 patients in its clinic database (https://weinbergcpcenter.org/research/cerebral-palsy-patient-registry/) and Nationwide Children's Hospital in Columbus, Ohio, which has set up their clinic as the Learn From Every Patient (LFEP) project.[5] There are several important CP registries outside the United States in Canada, Australia, Europe (Surveillance of Cerebral Palsy in Europe), and other locations.

Registries are powerful tools to investigate important clinical questions. They have limitations, in that they do not establish effectiveness the way that randomized controlled trials do. They also have their own unique issues related to recruitment, ethical considerations, and proper design.[3,6,7] The large number of patients entered into a registry, however, allows for techniques, such as practice-based evidence (PBE), to compare the effectiveness of different interventions in homogenous subgroups of patients (comparative effectiveness research [CER]). PBE research has addressed the shortcomings of previous research designs by developing a methodology that can handle multiple differences in CP treatments resulting from a large number of therapists and clinicians, at diverse sites, customizing many aspects of their treatment program, and treating patients with various levels of disability.[8] PBE studies have the following characteristics:

- They are prospective, multisite observational studies that capture practice variations existing both between and within sites.
- Sites enroll large numbers of consecutively treated patients, which permits analysis of subgroups of patients and cross-validation of findings.
- Treatment data are either abstracted from the medical record or provided by point-of-care documentation of therapies that are given during each surgical or

treatment session. Additional data may be collected through downloads of, for example, medication information.

- Outcome data are abstracted from the medical record, supplemented with information obtained from patient or caregiver interviews after various spans of time post-treatment.
- Clinicians and patients/caregivers often work together, which partially closes the circle of knowledge translation: clinicians and patients/caregivers are involved in initial design through final dissemination.
- The infrastructure created in a registry for PBE studies allow for the development of a learning health system, which informs and improves care with a continuing flow of data input, analysis, and practice improvement.[5]

Various experts have argued whether PBE studies can prove efficacy of treatment alternatives or whether their findings need to be confirmed by randomized controlled trials (RCTs). However this question is viewed, one conclusion is clear: PBE studies are superior to RCTs when it comes to external validity (generalizability): (1) placebos are replaced by real-life treatments (eg, alternative approaches being used by clinicians); (2) narrowly defined patient samples using multiple inclusion/exclusion criteria are replaced by a sample including every patient/caregiver who consents to be observed (and because there are no required treatment regimens that may pose varying risks, most patients consent or consent is waivered); and (3) surrogate outcome measures are replaced by real-life outcomes (eg, function, participation, long-term use of health care resources). Thus, PBE studies address all the requirements of well-designed CER. Findings have the potential to influence decisions of patients, caregivers, clinicians, and administrators.

The CPRN provides an illustration of the development, utility, and strength of a clinical network for CP. The CPRN hosts a multicenter clinical research registry for CP across the life span. The registry is augmented by patient-reported outcomes either gathered directly into the electronic health record (EHR) or from a community registry designed to be collected longitudinally. The impetus for the registry came from a workshop hosted by the National Institutes of Health (NIH) in 2014 entitled "State-of-the-Science and Treatment Decisions in Cerebral Palsy," which was designed to examine critical gaps in evidence and treatment of individuals with varying forms of CP[9] (see **Fig. 1**). The workshop highlighted numerous knowledge gaps, in particular a need for detailed information about types, timing, and intensity of interventions and patient factors associated with the best longitudinal outcomes.[9] Afterward, a group of stakeholders met to discuss the institution of a clinical, health condition–based multicenter registry for CP. The group included expertise in clinical practice, clinical research, biostatistics, epidemiology, and information technology as well as family members of individuals with CP. It formed into a task force supported by the NIH with coleaders Paul Gross, an Advisory Council member of the National Institute of Neurological Disorders and Stroke

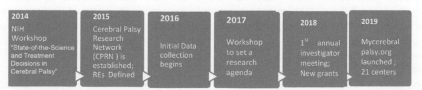

Fig. 1. Timeline of establishment and activities of the CPRN.

(NINDS), a cofounder of the Hydrocephalus Clinical Research Network, and a parent of a child with CP; and Deborah Gaebler-Spira, MD, a pediatric physiatrist at the Shirley Ryan AbilityLab in Chicago and former president of the American Academy for Cerebral Palsy and Developmental Medicine (AACPDM).

The group initiated a participatory action research process.[10] The steps involved were to listen, reflect, plan/analyze, and take action.

LISTEN

The goal of the listen phase was to gather feedback on the purpose, content, and structure of a registry. Consumers, advocates, researchers, and clinicians participated in consensus building through an iterative process that included recorded webinars, face-to-face and virtual meetings, online surveys, and sessions at professional meetings. More than 100 individuals provided input and feedback. Participants emphasized that the registry should harness the power of the EHR quantify practice variation, facilitate quality-improvement (QI) initiatives, support hypothesis generation for clinical research, and track outcomes across the International Classification of Functioning, Disability and Health (ICF) for individuals with CP. The registry should facilitate prospective multicenter CER to address a high priority question: Which interventions, including surgeries, injections, medications, and therapies lead to better functional and participatory outcomes across the various clinical presentations (Gross Motor Function Classification System [GMFCS] levels, age, etc), and other health characteristics?

REFLECT

In the reflect phase, participants/stakeholders reviewed existing national and international registries for CP and other rare diseases for (1) their content; (2) whether and how they interfaced with consumers and clinicians; and (3) successful examples of sustainable business models. This critical analysis of current registries informed the role, purpose, and structure of a new clinical registry for CP and would help to determine logistics of data management, storage, and sustainability. The group also looked for information technology strategies that would allow for flexibility to modify data elements over time and to leverage multiple EHR platforms. Along with existing CP registries, several other clinical registries were examined, including the Vermont Oxford Network,[11] the Hydrocephalus Clinical Research Network,[12] the Childhood Arthritis and Rheumatology Research Alliance,[13] and others that provided examples for clinical research and quality-improvement studies using registries as well as examples of patient-reported outcomes.

Funding models were examined. Registry projects could not expect funding from federal agencies, such as the NIH or Centers for Disease Control and Prevention,[14] so other strategies were used, including participation fees, institutional support, and philanthropic funding. The Nationwide Children's Hospital LFEP project was an example of a registry/learning health system that started with philanthropic funding and then received hospital support. The LFEP had demonstrated its value for improving care.[5] It was designed to have data collection as a part of routine clinical care using Epic (Verona, Wisconsin) EHR forms designed by the clinical team and to have the data transferred to the clinical note. This methodology not only facilitated research and quality improvement but also saved time and decreased clinician documentation burden.

The reflection process led to a vision to create a multi-institution, clinical research registry. Some of the primary principles learned from this process included (1) designing the registry to be woven into everyday clinical practice and not increase clinician burden; (2) leveraging the EHR for data collection; (3) focusing the registry on clinical care of the individual with CP; and (4) the importance of patient-reported outcomes. In order to succeed, there would need to be a consensus on goals and registry elements (REs) across the institutions involved.

PLAN/ANALYZE

The plan/analyze phase was designed to create a consensus on discrete items to include in the REs. The ICF framework[15] was a guide for determining the scope of the REs. Four work groups were established to develop REs: (1) nonsurgical physicians (developmental pediatricians, physiatrists, and neurologists); (2) orthopedic surgeons; (3) neurosurgeons; (4) and physical therapists, occupational therapists, and speech therapists. Each group had 8 to 11 members. An adult work group of 14 members was created to vet all items for applicability across the lifespan. A biostatistician (Susan Horn, PhD) supported the work and participated in the calls. Web-based tools were used to allow communication within and between groups and to keep the process open and transparent. Over 18 months, each work group came to consensus about the REs related to their discipline, which led to variation between groups. For example, tone measurements included Ashworth Scale, Modified Ashworth Scale, or Tardieu Scale, depending on the group. A set of parent/patient-reported therapy questions was created to gather information about recent use of equipment and therapy services, including place of service. The neurosurgeon work group focused on 2 surgical interventions—the intrathecal baclofen pump and selective dorsal rhizotomy. The group emphasized factors used in surgical decision making, intraoperative variables, and typical postoperative data collected in clinic. The orthopedic work group examined differences in intervention based on GMFCS level. Ambulatory patients (GMFCS I–III) generally had procedures to improve gait. For GMFCS IV–V, hip surveillance was a critical issue, and the group adopted the case report forms that had been developed for an international multi-institution cohort study of hip interventions in CP.[16] The work group also reviewed data fields collected in the registry at the Nemours Alfred I. duPont Hospital for Children. In order to simplify and focus the initial iteration of the registry, the work group decided to limit data collection to surgeries of the lower extremities and to leave upper extremity and spinal interventions for the future.

After completion of the initial efforts of each work group, there was a cross-group review to provide feedback, suggest changes, and harmonize items as much as possible. The statistical team de-duplicated items and developed Web forms using Research Electronic Data Capture, which provided a formal data dictionary for the REs and a visual representation of the registry. The REs contains 933 data items over the 4 disciplinary areas. The REs were cross-referenced with the first version of the NINDS CP common data elements (CDEs). There was an overlap of 221 items between the NINDS CDEs and the REs. The nonoverlapping elements were generally related to interventions or patient clinical characteristics that were not part of the NINDS effort. The groups determined that over time more effort would be made to match NINDS CDEs in the CPRN database and also made recommendations to the NINDS CDE committee to make some changes.

ACTION

The action phase involved launching the registry. In 2015, the leaders of the clinical registry and the 4 disciplinary work groups, a consumer representative, and the biostatistical lead established the CPRN and formed its initial executive committee.

The University of Utah was chosen to create and manage the registry with the support of philanthropic funding. Twenty-one institutions were initial members, representing the diversity of disciplines and geographic locations. Each institution made an application to its institutional review boards and initiated a business associate agreement with the University of Utah. Initial data collection occurred at Nationwide Children's Hospital in 2016. In the fall of 2017, CPRN extended an open invitation for institutions to join the registry on its Web site at http://cprn.org/join. There are now 23 participating centers and more in the process of considering membership (**Table 1**).

Community participation is a founding principle of CPRN. To this end, CPRN has community advisory boards both for parents of children with CP and for adults who have CP. The boards participate in discussion about the directions of CPRN and are asked to give input into projects proposing to use the CRPN infrastructure. In order to better inform the research goals for CPRN, and for the field in general, CPRN (Paul Gross) joined with the advocacy group CP NOW (Michele Shusterman) to obtain a grant from the Patient-Centered Outcomes Research Institute to develop a patient-centered research agenda for CP. This effort, which became known as Research CP, brought together clinicians, researchers, advocates, policy makers, and people with CP and their caregivers to put forth research priorities, based on the concept of "nothing about us without us."[17] Research CP used a community-based participatory approach combined with education and consensus building activities. There were 4 steps: (1) conduct a series of online webinars to educate interested participants about clinical research related to CP, including design,

Table 1
Participating clinical centers (as of 2019)

Hospital/University	Location
Nemours Alfred I. duPont Hospital for Children	Wilmington, Delaware
Boston Children's/Harvard Medical School	Boston, Massachusetts
Children's Hospital Colorado/University of Colorado	Denver Colorado
Children's of Alabama/University of Alabama	Birmingham, Alabama
Children's Mercy Hospital/University of Missouri-Kansas City	Kansas City, Missouri
Gillette Children's Specialty Healthcare	St. Paul, Minnesota
Michigan Medicine/University of Michigan	Ann Arbor, Michigan
Nationwide Children's Hospital/Ohio State University	Columbus, Ohio
Primary Children's Hospital/University of Utah	Salt Lake City, Utah
Rady Children's Hospital/University of California, San Diego	San Diego, California
Riley Children's Hospital/Indiana University	Indianapolis, Indiana
Scottish Rite Children's Hospital	Atlanta, Georgia
Seattle Children's Hospital/University of Washington	Seattle, Washington
Texas Children's Hospital/Baylor College of Medicine	Houston, Texas
UCLA Health/UCSF	Los Angeles, California
UCSF Benioff Children's Hospital Oakland	Oakland, California
UF Health/University of Florida	Jacksonville, Florida
UNC Medical Center/University of North Carolina–Chapel Hill	Chapel Hill, North Carolina
University of Texas Health Science Center–Houston	Houston, Texas
UVA Health System/University of Virginia	Charlottesville, Virginia
Yale-New Haven Hospital/Yale University	New Haven, Connecticut

funding, and similar issues; (2) use a Web-based mechanism to generate research ideas and create consensus; (3) set the research agenda at workshop with representatives of all of the stakeholders; and (4) disseminate the findings through publication and presentation.

The webinar series had 275 participants recruited from advocacy organizations, the AACPDM, and social media. After the first webinar, participants were invited to contribute to an iterative online process via Codigital Ltd. This online external crowdsourcing intermediary provides a platform for participants to record ideas, and then edit and vote on the ideas of others. Using this method, 392 ideas were generated with 26,798 votes cast. The leadership team of Research CP, which consisted of consumers, researchers, and clinicians, participated in a Delphi process to evaluate the list of the highest-priority research ideas and create a workable, less redundant list for the next phase. Ideas that suggested advocacy and education projects or clinical guideline development were not included because the leadership group felt that they deserved a different avenue of consideration. The 20 highest ranking ideas were presented to the workshop.

Workshop participants were chosen by the leadership group based on engagement in the process up to that point; diversity by geography, race, gender, and other participant factors (for professionals, of discipline, seniority, and clinical/research distribution of their career; for consumers, of age and clinical factors); and of availability. There were 47 participants, a science writer, and a facilitator. The participants were asked to further clarify the ideas and to share thoughts and observations about the experience. In the end, 16 research ideas were prioritized into an agenda (**Table 2**). Life span issues and longitudinal studies were highly prioritized as were more investigation into symptoms, such as pain and fatigue. Comparative effectiveness of interventions and exercise fitness and health also ranked high. The participants expressed a strong appreciation for the value of engagement between consumers, clinicians, and researchers. They also placed an emphasis on outcomes that looked at participation in the community more so than physical measures.

CPRN formalized its structure, establishing committees related to scientific and article review, and standard operating procedures for its functions. CPRN first reported its registry findings on the first 829 patients in September 2017 at the annual meeting of the AACPDM and again in October 2018, with 2074 patients.

In June of 2018, CPRN held its first investigators meeting in Houston, Texas. At that meeting, CPRN reviewed the Research CP agenda and measured its current project pipeline against it. It found that there were several CER projects in place and in the pipeline, but there needed to be more work on longitudinal projects and work related to fitness and risk of chronic disease. Some of the more prominent current projects discussed at the meeting included proposals to add the study of epilepsy to the network and to gather search for genetic causes of CP. Both of these study areas were subsequently funded by the Pediatric Epilepsy Research Foundation and the NINDS. In addition, the focus on filling gaps in a patient-centered research agenda has led to the creation of several additional study groups developing proposals for research to address these gaps.

In August 2018, CPRN's first article on the results of its Research CP initiative was published in *Developmental Medicine and Child Neurology*[17]. Its presence at the annual meeting of AACPDM has grown from 3 abstracts in 2017 to 8 for 2019 as its registry and other research efforts begin to produce preliminary findings.

CPRN has established a need and a solution for clinical registry data to address critical questions in the care and treatment of CP. It has coupled these clinical data

Table 2	
Top sixteen research ideas	
Number	**Research Idea**
1	Research the issues around aging with CP, not only to understand how to treat adults now but also to update treatments and therapies with children who have CP to prevent some of the secondary impairments, such as pain, fatigue, and functional loss.
2	What are the best long-term exercise/strength training strategies to improve activity, participation and health, minimize pain, and maximize function in each GMFCS category across the life span?
3	Which interventions (surgeries, injections, medications, and therapies [orthotics, equipment, and training]) are associated with better functional outcomes (important to child/family) controlling for GMFCS level, age, and comorbidities?
4	Increasing age is related to pain and fatigue in people with CP, regardless of GMFCS level. What variables are important to monitor/treat early on in life to prevent the development of pain and fatigue later on in life?
5	What are the best methods and ways to reduce pain, falling, lack of stamina, and deterioration of function that can have a negative impact on the quality of life for people with CP especially in adulthood?
6	Research effective ways to build and maintain strength, flexibility, and endurance health in children and adults with CP. How can better ways be found to successfully integrate these into daily living?
7	Develop and test effective methods for exercise and increased physical activity for individuals who are less ambulatory (some GMFCS III, and GMFCS IV and V), including techniques, proper dosing, and information on effects on strength and health.
8	How can the brain's neuroplasticity be best leveraged to retrain neural pathways for improved motor function, speech function, and mobility?
9	Have large-scale studies that follow children with the various types of CP throughout adulthood to discover how the aging process affects individuals with different types of CP and severity levels.
10	What are effective treatment methods to address differential outcomes in adolescents and adults related to pain, fatigue, and early functional loss?
11	Study the outcomes of complementary and nontraditional therapies (hyperbaric oxygen, hippotherapy, swimming/aquatic, Feldenkrais, massage, yoga, tai chi, music, recreational, acupuncture, and so forth), reviewing efficacy, costs, insurance support probabilities.
12	Research the effectiveness of intensive physical therapy programs, bursts of services, combined protocols (eg, botulinum toxin with intensive physical therapy, constraint therapy with robotics, etc). Evidence of efficacy is needed to get ALL insurers to fully cover the treatment options that work.
13	How are functional independence and life participation of children and adults with CP best maximized?
14	Identify biomarkers (neuroimaging, blood, cerebrospinal fluid, and amniotic fluid) to help determine which individuals respond best to which interventions (therapy, medical, and surgical) so that treatment approaches can be tailored to each individual person with CP.
15	Quality of life is an important goal for several questions related to CP. How is it quantified that to really answer which interventions produce the greatest benefit to quality of life?
16	Not much work has been done on the cognitive impairments, including difficulties with math and any subject with spatial orientation.

Adapted from Gross PH, Bailes AF, Horn SD, et al. Setting a patient-centered research agenda for cerebral palsy: a participatory action research initiative. Dev Med Child Neurol. 2018;60(12):1282; with permission.

with complementary patient-reported outcomes data with an infrastructure that enables the longitudinal following of this population to answer fundamental questions about how childhood interventions affect long-term functional mobility, participation, and quality of life. CPRN needs to establish an entity structure by which it can garner funds to sustain its operations and pursue additional grant funding for its research. This step will allow CPRN to establish itself as a network of learning health systems that use its registry as a platform for continuous improvement in the outcomes for people with cerebral palsy—not only generating the evidence for the best practices but also measuring their implementation and impact at hospitals throughout North America.

REFERENCES

1. Kirby RS, Wingate MS, Van Naarden Braun K, et al. Prevalence and functioning of children with cerebral palsy in four areas of the United States in 2006: a report from the Autism and Developmental Disabilities Monitoring Network. Res Dev Disabil 2011;32(2):462–9.
2. Villamor E, Tedroff K, Peterson M, et al. Association between maternal body mass index in early pregnancy and incidence of cerebral palsy. JAMA 2017;317(9): 925–36.
3. Hogan DB, Warner J, Patten S, et al. Ethical and legal considerations for Canadian registries. Can J Neurol Sci 2013;40(Suppl 2):S5–23.
4. Lyu H, Cooper M, Patel K, et al. Prevalence and data transparency of National Clinical Registries in the United States. J Healthc Qual 2016;38(4):223–34.
5. Lowes LP, Noritz GH, Newmeyer A, et al. 'Learn from every patient': implementation and early results of a learning health system. Dev Med Child Neurol 2017; 59(2):183–91.
6. Hamilton M, Genge A, Johnston M, et al. Patient recruitment by Neurological Registries. Can J Neurol Sci 2013;40(Suppl 2):S23–6.
7. Pringsheim T, Marrie RA, Donner E, et al. Neurological Registry feasibility and sustainability. Can J Neurol Sci 2013;40(Suppl. 2):S55–9.
8. Horn SD, DeJong G, Deutscher D. Practice-based evidence research in rehabilitation: an alternative to randomized controlled trials and traditional observational studies. Arch Phys Med Rehabil 2012;93(8 Suppl):S127–37.
9. Lungu C, Hirtz D, Damiano D, et al. Report of a workshop on research gaps in the treatment of cerebral palsy. Neurology 2016;87(12):1293–8.
10. Baum F, MacDougall C, Smith D. Participatory action research. J Epidemiol Community Health 2006;60(10):854–7.
11. Network, V.O. Vermont Oxford Network: about us 2017. 2017. Available at: https:// public.vtoxford.org/about-us/. Accessed April 12, 2019.
12. Simon TD, Hall M, Riva-Cambrin J, et al. Infection rates following initial cerebrospinal fluid shunt placement across pediatric hospitals in the United States. Clinical article. J Neurosurg Pediatr 2009;4(2):156–65.
13. Sandborg C. The future of rheumatology research: the Childhood Arthritis and Rheumatology Research Alliance. Curr Probl Pediatr Adolesc Health Care 2006;36(3):104–9.
14. Wu YW, Mehravari AS, Numis AL, et al. Cerebral palsy research funding from the National Institutes of Health, 2001 to 2013. Dev Med Child Neurol 2015;57(10): 936–41.
15. World Health Organization. International classification of functioning, disability and health (ICF). Geneva (Switzerland): World Health Organization; 2001.

16. Dobson F, Boyd RN, Parrott J, et al. Hip surveillance in children with cerebral palsy. Impact on the surgical management of spastic hip disease. J Bone Joint Surg Br 2002;84(5):720–6.

17. Gross PH, Bailes AF, Horn SD, et al. Setting a patient-centered research agenda for cerebral palsy: a participatory action research initiative. Dev Med Child Neurol 2018;60(12):1278–84.

Moving?

Make sure your subscription moves with you!

To notify us of your new address, find your **Clinics Account Number** (located on your mailing label above your name), and contact customer service at:

Email: journalscustomerservice-usa@elsevier.com

800-654-2452 (subscribers in the U.S. & Canada)
314-447-8871 (subscribers outside of the U.S. & Canada)

Fax number: 314-447-8029

Elsevier Health Sciences Division
Subscription Customer Service
3251 Riverport Lane
Maryland Heights, MO 63043

*To ensure uninterrupted delivery of your subscription, please notify us at least 4 weeks in advance of move.

Printed and bound by CPI Group (UK) Ltd, Croydon, CR0 4YY

03/10/2024

01040403-0020